THE TRAUMA
OF BURNOUT

Dr. Claire Plumbly is a clinical psychologist and director of Good Therapy Ltd, a trauma-focused therapy practice based online and in Taunton, UK.

Claire has over twenty years of experience working therapeutically with individuals suffering with anxiety, trauma, and burnout, both in the National Health Service and private practice. She is also an accredited cognitive behavioral therapy (CBT) practitioner and eye movement desensitization and reprocessing (EMDR) consultant-supervisor. Connect with Claire on social media: @drclaireplumbly.

THE TRAUMA OF BURNOUT

How to Manage Your Nervous System
Before It Manages You

DR. CLAIRE PLUMBLY

balance

New York   Boston

Copyright © 2025 by Claire Plumbly
Cover design by Terri Sirma
Cover image by Mike Flippo/Shutterstock
Cover copyright © 2025 by Hachette Book Group, Inc.

Published in Great Britain as *Burnout: How to Manage Your Nervous System Before It Manages You* in 2024 by Yellow Kite, an imprint of Hodder & Stoughton, a Hachette UK company.

The author is grateful to the copyright holders who have granted permission to reproduce extracts from their work, as listed on the following pages: 6, 99, 148, 167, 183, 192, 220, and 234.

Diagrams redrawn by Craig Burgess

Balance
Hachette Book Group
1290 Avenue of the Americas
New York, NY 10104
GCP-Balance.com
@GCPBalance

First Edition: January 2025

Balance is an imprint of Grand Central Publishing. The Balance name and logo are registered trademarks of Hachette Book Group, Inc.

The publisher is not responsible for websites (or their content) that are not owned by the publisher.

The Hachette Speakers Bureau provides a wide range of authors for speaking events. To find out more, visit hachettespeakersbureau.com or email HachetteSpeakers@hbgusa.com.

Balance books may be purchased in bulk for business, educational, or promotional use. For information, please contact your local bookseller or email the Hachette Book Group Special Markets Department at Special.Markets@hbgusa.com.

Typeset in Celeste by Hewer Text UK Ltd, Edinburgh

Library of Congress Cataloging-in-Publication Data has been applied for.

ISBNs: 978-0-306-83631-2 (trade paperback); 978-0-306-83632-9 (ebook)

Printed in the United States of America

LSC-C

Printing 1, 2024

CONTENTS

CONTENTS

AUTHOR'S NOTE

In this book I have distilled and simplified key research into burnout, but please keep in mind that burnout manifests differently for different people. If one of these ideas does not resonate, the fact that it is still a broad concept, with different measurements and sometimes even definitions, could be the reason. Burnout interventions can be directed at different levels including the individual, team, organization, and society. A book addressing all of these at once would be enormous. This book is aimed at the individual level, in particular, for those with overwhelmed nervous systems who feel stuck.

Throughout the book I illustrate points with stories. These are based on an amalgamation of clients I've worked with over many years, or other people in my life. I have changed the names and identifying details such as gender, profession, and situation to protect identities and confidentiality. Where specific situations have been drawn upon to exemplify a point, I have been given consent to do so.

The neuroscience described in this book is designed to give you language and concepts that can help you to make sense of your experiences so they feel less intimidating and understandable. However, neuroscience is a complex field to draw from, so this book simplifies concepts from the research to make them as accessible as possible for the subject of burnout.

Remember to take into account any injuries or illnesses that may not make these individual exercises suitable. If you are unsure please consult your physician.

A last but important point: This book is not intended to replace professional help. If you are struggling with your well-being, please consider seeking further support from a mental-health professional or your doctor to get an assessment and personalized plan of support.

INTRODUCTION

For more than an hour before her alarm sounded, Sarah had stared at the ceiling mentally working on projects. But, despite having been awake for so long, it took all her might to force her body up from the bed. It felt heavy, not properly rested, and her mind felt as if it had never switched off, with thoughts jumping haphazardly between things she had to do, and failing to settle on any one of them for long enough to form a plan. She went through the motions of getting washed and dressed, then found herself downstairs. She headed into the living room—but what had she come in here for? This kept happening. For weeks, she hadn't been able to stay focused on things. As she trudged toward the front door, passing all the half-finished jobs that lay scattered about the house, her partner called.

"Sar, could you pick up dinner on your way home tonight?"

Another demand… Why always me? Everyone seems to need a piece of me all the time. Then, a painful wave of anxiety flooded her as she remembered what happened yesterday. She shouldn't have snapped at that student who'd asked when the grades would be in. She wished she hadn't done that. What if they made a complaint? *It's just there's too much to do and never enough time.* Her phone lit up. Oh no, another message from Alison, a good friend. Damn, she never got back to her last time. But she didn't have time now. Work was just too busy and demanding to think beyond it to anything else.

To her colleagues, Sarah appeared to be her usual diligent self, but underneath she felt flat and demotivated. Her lesson plans had shrunk to scant one-liners. She was busier than ever but without the enthusiasm that used to fuel her. Reluctantly, she had plucked up the courage to tell the department manager: "I'm just feeling overwhelmed, really. A bit overstretched."

"But this is what the job entails, Sarah, I'm afraid. Would you like HR to send you some advice on time management?"

Instead of helping, this had knocked her confidence and she was left feeling like a failure. So this was it. With no one left to turn to, she felt trapped and alone.

Over time, Sarah spent more and more waking hours—and many of what should have been sleeping hours—playing catch-up. She did her grading while watching TV, worked late into the evening, and spent her lunchtime lesson-planning instead of eating or socializing with colleagues; chatting wasted precious time.

In the end, she wasn't doing anything at all for pleasure, and she laughed cynically when others talked of weekend outings and indulgences or hobbies. She maintained that it was because she didn't have time, but she had actually lost her ability to experience joy in these things and couldn't even remember why she used to enjoy them. She had become detached from those around her and couldn't imagine feeling any different.

At night, in bed, she'd get stuck scrolling on her phone, trying to escape the buzz of worrisome thoughts and the to-do list in her head. Her body was permanently tense, so that when she finally slept she would drift in and out of consciousness rather than sleeping deeply...

HOW BURNOUT IS DIFFERENT FROM STRESS

When our personal and work lives are relentlessly demanding, we become stretched. Like an elastic band, we have the capacity to stretch quite some way—in fact, stress can be a positive, healthy experience when there's the right amount, when we feel in control, and, importantly, when it has an end point. But when stress is inescapable, then we are stretched to maximum for too long, causing our nervous systems to get stuck in survival mode. The impact of this on our emotions, thoughts, body, and behaviors is the experience of burnout.

Many people struggle to notice just how stretched they have become and may assume that burnout refers to a complete breakdown (the band snapping); but in fact, being chronically overstretched affects our ability to function. Take Sarah, forgetting why she's walked into a room, snapping at students, and struggling to complete a thought. Dimly aware that she wasn't functioning well, that she was irritable and forgetful, but not at the point of awareness that she was burned out. (This is why I provide the progression of stress into burnout in Chapter 1—to help identify the stages.)

Burnout goes beyond healthy stress. When we are stressed, our reactions become busy and urgent, because our nervous systems are mobilized for action. We may get anxious or problem-focused thoughts as our brains work hard to find solutions. Burnout happens when we haven't found the solutions before we've completely spent our energy and resources looking for them. Essentially, healthy stress is an energized experience, where we are absorbed by reaching goals or "fixing" problems, whereas burnout is often a hollow experience of feeling we've given all we have and are now running on empty. Like Sarah, we might start to operate at an autopilot level, appearing to get stuff done but with no zest for life or the level of effectiveness we're truly capable of.

In burnout, we can feel emotionally blunted, cynical, unsure of ourselves, and detached from the people and activities that used to light us up. Moreover, burnout traps us in a cycle, believing we will feel calmer and safer if we can keep going and come out the other end; but *there is no end* and this thinking pattern just leads to functional decline, until, eventually, the brain or body forces a stop for us in the form of physical or mental illness or both.

Because the process of functional decline occurs gradually, it's hard during the early stages to spot signs that you are burning out. Boundaries are increasingly crossed; all the little crevasses of life once reserved for downtime get filled with "doing"; values are eroded or abandoned; and your sense of agency is lost. Not only do you stop enjoying life, but you also feel as though you are just going through the motions and have lost your sense of identity. On reaching this state of burnout, the nervous system's response makes it much harder for you to problem-solve, make rational decisions, and generally do the self-care you so desperately need. When you are in this state, you know you should be caring for yourself, but you can't seem to initiate or stay committed to this because you don't have the physical or mental resources. As a clinical psychologist, I've seen hundreds of clients with nervous systems affected this way by chronic stress.

WHY BURNOUT IS ENDEMIC TO MODERN LIFE

This type of human distress was first recognized when German-American psychologist Herbert Freudenberger coined the term "burnout" in 1974 to refer to the impact of work where it had placed "excessive demands on energy, strength or resources." Google searches for the term "burnout" have steadily increased as it's become an issue within a wide range of arenas: teacher burnout; academic burnout; entrepreneurial burnout; student burnout; parent burnout; health workers and therapists falling ill themselves or leaving their jobs because they were too burned out to carry on. A wildfire of burnout raging through society. But what caused it to spread?

In *Can't Even: How Millennials Became the Burnout Generation* journalist Anne Helen Petersen explores the historical cultural influences and power abuses that lead us to overwork. The American Dream perpetuates the myth of achieving rags to riches with hard work alone. Protestant ideals are woven into many Western values with hard work as proof of devotion. In modern times, we glorify work as only being worthwhile if you *love* it, leading to the acceptance of low-paid jobs that reward you in other ways regardless of how this affects your living standards and long-term future. And the impact of the pandemic, recession, and political unrest has generated a fear of losing it all.

These cultural influences fuel the sense that we shouldn't take our foot off the gas. We internalize the message that constant productiveness is a way to stay safe, earn our self-worth, and secure our social status, making it difficult or impossible to set boundaries around self-care and personal time. My clients often say they don't know where to start when I ask them about setting boundaries. It's not a skill that's being nurtured or modeled anywhere. Burnout is "a disease of civilization," according to the author and philosopher Pascal Chabot in his book *Global Burnout*, published in 2018. He sees civilization, having exploited our natural resources for many years, now proceeding to exhaust human resources, too.

And with an always-on, workaholic society comes a constant barrage of stimuli, pressure, decisions, commitments, and considerations. We used to talk about leaving our work at the office. Now we can work anywhere and always, and we do. This means that the human nervous system, equipped to cope with small-scale stimuli at intervals, is now being overwhelmed by thousands of stimuli per day.

What's more, modern life has interrupted our methods of resetting our nervous systems, too, by disconnecting from each other and our environments. Not only is the pace of life fast and furious, but it's more often conducted on screens. The opportunities for anchoring and settling our nervous systems are disappearing.

CAN YOU BE OFFICIALLY DIAGNOSED WITH BURNOUT?

In Britain, the dominant approach to understanding emotional distress is through the International Classification of Diseases (ICD), where patterns in behaviors are given diagnostic labels, like depression, generalized anxiety disorder, and so on. At the time of writing, the most recent edition of the ICD (the ICD-11) classifies "burnout" as a syndrome* "caused by chronic workplace stress that has not been successfully managed," while in the equivalent American manual, known as the *Diagnostic and Statistical Manual of Mental Disorders, 5th Edition* (DSM-5), there is no reference to it. The World Health Organization's (WHO) definition stems from the ICD-11, and they are clear that this is an "occupational phenomenon," rather than a medical condition.

There are countries where burnout has a formal status in clinical settings (France, Denmark, Sweden, for example) but in the US, UK, and Australia "burnout" is not routinely being recorded in patient notes. Physisicans are more likely to code a patient presenting with burnout-like difficulties as "stress at work," or label them with an anxiety or depression disorder instead.

The "occupational phenomenon" wording of the definition has meant that the term burnout has often been reserved for formal workplace settings only. But this restrictive understanding of work invalidates the experiences of billions of unpaid people, such as caregivers, parents, students, and so on, which itself has a negative impact on mental health. "Burnout" must no

---

*A syndrome is not a disease. It is a set of physical, emotional, or behavioral signs and complaints that appear alongside each other, creating a state that is out of the norm.

longer be left in the realm of occupational health where it first began. The physical, emotional, and behavioral difficulties described in burnout syndrome are issues that many people relate to, and, if they are left in this state without intervention, there can be serious implications for physical and mental health.

A second difficulty with the WHO definition is this: When are any of us "at work"? Unpaid work is part of *everyone's* life in some capacity, such as parenting or home chores. This is often experienced as that heart-sinking feeling of starting the "second shift" the moment you get home from work—all the tedious home-based duties, cooking, and laundry. Although this is not true of all relationships, research shows that females often end up doing the lion's share of this unpaid work, not just practically but also in terms of carrying the "mental load"—remembering to put items on the shopping list and sending a card for Grannie's birthday—which adds significantly to the exhaustion and the difficulty in switching off in the supposedly "safe" space of their own home.

Those self-identifying with burnout or those out sick with "stress" may not think to approach a mental-health specialist, but, contrary to popular belief, you don't need a formal mental-health diagnosis to seek support from a psychologist or mental-health professional. I hope this book will be a support to you or anyone who is feeling this way, providing ideas for coping and also a sense of what therapy could look like should you choose to get extra help.

ABOUT MY APPROACH

All clinical psychologists are trained in theories of human emotions and behavior that have been shown in research to be effective. These theories give us a framework that we use to carry out our work, from conducting therapy to writing a self-help book, and the ones we gravitate toward reflect our worldview as well as the needs of our client group.

As a psychologist specializing in trauma, I am drawn to trauma-informed theories—those that make sense of an individual's behavioral patterns and emotional distress in terms of what has happened to them, how this has set off their human survival responses, and what they need to do to cope with these events (which can cause internal pressures that contribute to burnout). This includes:

- past experiences that you may already have heard about; some examples from your recent past might be: a relationship ending; a restructure at work; a difficult boss at work; or the impact of experiences that go back further, such as having overly strict parents, being bullied, or having a lot of upheaval in your life
- pressures that occurred in your life that are less visible or obvious to you—things like expectations placed on you by your family of origin or society, your early relationships with your primary caregivers, inequalities, disempowerment, or unmet human needs.

When I'm in therapy with people, part of the work is to look out for both the visible and less visible experiences, explore how these were felt as threats, and help them understand how their negative emotional reactions and coping strategies therefore make sense. There is often relief on recognizing how an apparently innocuous event left a scar that has lasted into adulthood.

In recent years, there has been a trend in psychology, particularly in the field of trauma, toward listening more closely to the wisdom of our bodies and allowing that to guide us in what we need. If we listen and help the body to feel safe, this can trickle upward to bring the calmer thoughts and feelings that many who come to therapy are seeking. This book embraces this approach and there are two models I draw on most throughout. The first is Stephen W. Porges' polyvagal theory (PVT), which helps us to see what's happening to the nervous system in chronic stress. An understanding of this fuels motivation to practice the self-care tools regularly which brings change more quickly. (The original nervous-system model of stress for psychotherapy was based on only two branches of the nervous system: the parasympathetic or green mode and sympathetic or amber mode. While this can explain some of the problems in burnout, like frenetic and irritable difficulties, PVT's description of a third dorsal vagal branch gives us extra language to understand how shut down and hopeless many people feel in later-stage burnout.)

But burnout recovery isn't a quick fix. So to understand your nervous system in context, we will also draw on the wisdom of compassion-focused therapy (CFT). This not only provides a map of how you got stuck here but also a longer-term road out. By improving self-soothing and self-compassion, an embodied experience that stimulates the neural pathways related to feeling calm and connected to those around you, you build your capacity to stick with the self-care routines that you *know* will help you, yet you often overlook.

WHAT TO EXPECT IN THIS BOOK

I have based the structure of this book on the format psychologists tend to follow in therapy: assessment of your issues, the neuroscience you need to understand yourself, the provision of quick-start tools for regulating your nervous system, and then a deeper dive into the underlying patterns that keep repeating themselves and learning how to break out of these.

In Part 1 ("The Overwhelmed Nervous System—How It Stifles Your Ability to Think and Enjoy Life"), we look at the problems caused by burnout, how to recognize it at different stages, and how to spot it before it stops you in your tracks. I also show why burnout traps you and alters your behavior, your emotions, and your perspective, before explaining the physiological reasons for these changes. Part 1 ends with Chapter 5, which gives tools for quickly regulating a frazzled nervous system.

Part 2 ("The Forces That Drive Us Toward Burnout—and How We Get Stuck There") explains how it's not your fault that you burn out. It shows how to develop a framework for understanding thought patterns, habits, and behaviors that promote burnout based on past experiences and present-day difficulties. It helps you to see what to focus on to understand roadblocks so you can navigate them rather than allow them to derail you completely.

Part 3 ("Rebalancing to Recover from Burnout") shares ways to improve your self-compassion for longer-term healthy balance. I will also show you how to apply these ideas with the people around you.

Part 4 ("Post-Burnout Growth") gives you the steps for not only avoiding burnout in the future but also taking what you've learned from the negative experience of burning out and using it to grow and thrive and protect yourself in the future.

Throughout the book I use case studies based on an amalgamation of clients I have worked with over many years. Names have been changed and sometimes gender, profession, and situation, to protect the identities and confidentiality of these people. In particular, I focus on four characters who are all under stress at work and also present with internal pressures that we might typically work on in therapy when they are burned out. They are Anika (a senior nurse in a county hospital), Scott (an entrepreneur who has worked hard to build his business), Suraj (a junior architect who has a job in a well-regarded firm), and Sarah (a teacher who is off work due to stress).

The main message throughout this book is that burnout is not your fault; it is a combination of many factors, which we can tease out together here. Despite this, it is within your power to make positive changes—even small ones can have a big effect over time. And this book will show you how.

Part 1

THE OVERWHELMED NERVOUS SYSTEM— HOW IT STIFLES YOUR ABILITY TO THINK AND ENJOY LIFE

Imagine two people buy the same model of car. Both are equally good drivers, but the first person is a trained mechanic while the second has no clue when it comes to how cars work. When the cars start to make an intermittent clanging sound, the mechanic is attuned to what this could be and immediately pulls over to do checks and adjustments. The other driver does not notice the clanging at first, but when it does finally register in his awareness he just thinks hopefully, *Hmm that's irritating, I hope it goes away soon!*

Similarly, when we understand what's under our nervous-system bonnets and have the tools to do the necessary work, we can catch problems at the first sign of trouble. And Part 1 will teach you exactly that, giving you what you need in order to become your own mechanic for the human autonomic nervous system.

Chapter 1

HOW BURNOUT FEELS

———————

Anika came to me several months after being off work and out sick when she became physically unwell and started having panic attacks. She was a senior nurse on the ward who had gradually worked her way up the ladder. I asked her to describe her typical working day.

She told me she'd been getting up at 5:30 a.m. to clean the house before work and, at the end of her shift after the ward staff change when everyone else headed home, she had started returning to the ward, driven by a constant sense of guilt and duty and a need to finish whatever work she had started rather than hand over a half-completed job to a colleague. Inevitably, once she got back on the ward and sucked into doing new tasks, her colleagues would forget that she was working beyond her allotted shift. When she eventually arrived home, it was late in the evening. Her days ended as they began under the cover of darkness. The family had already eaten. She reheated dinner with no time left to relax and engage with her partner and children, and then she went to bed, exhausted. Her mind still buzzing, she lay in bed and picked up her phone, and, before she knew it, she'd purchased another five items of clothing she didn't need.

Anika referred to herself as a swan, paddling like mad under the water but seemingly calm above it. She'd grown so accustomed to the high level of stress and her overworking to compensate that she had lost sight of how stretched she was.

"I never felt I'd done all I could," she told me. "There was always more, so I didn't think I could stop. I didn't even have enough spare headspace for my partner and kids, to be honest. I lost touch with what they were up to. My work was all-consuming and I was preoccupied with the needs of my patients and making sure I didn't lose my job."

She moved through her home routines in a haze, and at work she was swept into the tide of emergencies, routine checks, and the endless stream of paperwork that marked her days. She was driven by a sense of duty and an ingrained belief that she was indispensable. The niggles of life, those small, persistent issues that once felt manageable, now loomed large, magnified by her weariness. The solace she used to find in organizing her space and clearing her inbox to give herself a sense of control amid the chaos no longer provided relief, and she had turned to quick-relief options that she knew were less healthy but she couldn't seem to rein in: drinking more alcohol, compulsive social media scrolling, or online shopping. It took several months off work for her to start feeling better, as her body gradually unfroze and climbed down from her stress and anxiety.

Why had Anika failed to see how stressed she was for so long? Why hadn't she been able to take a break before her body forced this upon her?

Anika's experiences matched with the three dimensions of occupational burnout, as defined by professor Christina Maslach, a social psychologist who became interested in the "detached concern" she was seeing in caregiving professionals and whose work has been foundational to our current conceptualization and measurement of burnout:

- **Physical and Emotional Exhaustion:** Feeling worn out, drained, or lethargic. You might feel heavy or sluggish, or emotionally as though you have nothing left to give. People in burnout often report feeling stressed and overwhelmed, irritable, or depressed. This can also develop into demotivation or reduced passion for work.

- **Feeling of Detachment (Referred to as Depersonalization):** An experience of disengaging from work or life, sometimes known as "compassion fatigue" or a more generalized difficulty in "feeling"—a numbness. This was what Maslach described as "detached concern," and it can also look like cynicism or emotional avoidance.

- **Reduced Personal Accomplishment or Sense of Ineffectiveness:** You may become less effective in what you're doing due to the aforementioned issues—for example, exhaustion and brain fog can make it hard to concentrate or think clearly. Higher procrastination may mean jobs are avoided, or rushing may cause mistakes. Cynicism and emotional exhaustion may mean that you do tasks but aren't paying close attention to detail or are cutting corners as a coping mechanism. You may also believe you are no good at what you do and be highly critical of your efforts and work.

Maslach's description is the basis of the current official definition by the World Health Organization. But her pioneering work has been added to by further research, published in 2021, by clinical psychiatrist Professor Gordon Parker and colleagues in Sydney, Australia. Their study of 1,019 participants self-identifying with burnout included people involved in paid work but also people in unpaid roles, such as parents and informal caregivers. From this, they created a list of the most frequently reported physical and emotional problems in burnout*:

- **Exhaustion** (cited by 69 percent of the sample)—experienced as fatigue, tiredness, lethargy, and feeling drained
- **Anxiety** (51 percent)—feeling stressed, worried, and overwhelmed, unable to relax or switch off, ruminating about work when not there, experiencing a sense of dread, and feeling fidgety or restless
- **Indifference** (47 percent)—experienced as a lack of empathy and interest or pleasure in work or activities outside of work, cynicism, apathy, disengagement, lack of feeling, and instead just "going through the motions"
- **Depression** (38 percent)—low mood and sadness, hopelessness and helplessness, lowered self-worth, self-doubt, and even (albeit rarely) suicidal thoughts
- **Irritability and Anger** (35 percent)—with frequent descriptors of this being impatience, agitation, frustration, and resentment
- **Sleep Disturbance** (34 percent)—with either lack of sleep or excessive sleep being reported
- **Lack of Motivation or Passion** (33 percent)—experienced as an absence of satisfaction in life and/or work, feelings of not making any difference at work, or that work lacks purpose or reduced passion for their job
- **Cognitive Problems** (32 percent)—including concentration, attention and memory problems, "brain fog" or cloudy thinking, difficulty in planning or making decisions, as well as feeling confused

---

*Data from the Sydney studies. Table of the 12 main symptoms volunteered by subjects about their burnout syndrome © 2022 Gordon Parker, Gabriela Tavella and Kerrie Eyers. Reproduced with permission of Taylor & Francis through PLSclear.

- **Impaired Performance** (26 percent)—evidenced by lower productivity, reduced quality of output, making more mistakes, avoiding responsibilities, and procrastinating
- **Becoming Asocial** (25 percent)—effectively cocooning and withdrawing from family, friends, colleagues, and clients
- **Physical Symptoms** (25 percent)—aches or headaches, eating and appetite changes, nausea, and low libido
- **Emotional Liability** (16 percent)—fragile emotions, increased sensitivity, and emotional outbursts and being more tearful

The reason for these common experiences is rooted in our nervous systems' response to prolonged, persistent stress. We will see why they respond like this and the relationship between trauma and burnout in the next two chapters. But first let's look at the common situations that cause us to burn out.

UNDERSTANDING COMPASSION FATIGUE

"Compassion fatigue" is a term you hear frequently in relation to the second dimension of burnout (a feeling of detachment), especially from people in caring professions who spend time with distressed individuals. However, many psychologists would argue that compassion cannot fatigue, and that, in fact, this term is related to empathy.

Empathy is characterized as feeling the positive or negative emotions of others. Being with others' emotional pain like this for a long time can, therefore, be tiring and overwhelming. Compassion, on the other hand, is a desire to make things better, with a warm, kind, and nonjudgmental approach. Self-compassion is responding in this way to your own distress. Empathy is one aspect of compassion, but on its own empathy is tiring and emotionally consuming. If you take on the distress of others without replenishing your

---

own emotional needs (using self-compassion), then this leads to overload which can depress your emotions and make you feel hopeless.

For this reason, "empathic distress fatigue" is a more accurate term for this experience.

THE TRIGGERS AND PATTERNS OF BURNOUT

Research by professor of psychology and education Barry Farber into therapist and teacher burnout led to findings that there are three dominant patterns of reacting to work-related stress— three subtypes of burnout (although he points out that we might oscillate between these at different times):

- Frenetic burnout
- Underchallenged burnout
- Worn-out burnout

The most commonly reported subtype is frenetic burnout, but many people I've worked with experience all three at once.

Let's look at each of them in turn.

Frenetic Burnout

This describes the pattern of working harder and harder in response to stress. It happens when the demands of work outweigh the resources needed to do it comfortably and there's an ambition to do it well. Your work–life boundaries therefore slip, and work becomes all encompassing. Those who care passionately about what they do are at higher risk of this, particularly where budget cuts and shrinking margins have led to a lack of staff, squeezing those who are left, and, as we will see in Chapter 7, there are social pressures on us to view this pattern of burnout as normal. The typical trajectory of this type of burnout tends to be high anxiety and irritability, followed by physical exhaustion, then emotional numbing to it all, leading to feeling less connected with your surroundings and then generally cynical. Staff who are new to their job or career are particularly susceptible to this type of burnout.

Underchallenged Burnout

Burnout doesn't just occur as a result of being overstretched. Monotonous work or work where there is no prospect of self-development is understimulating. If you carry out repetitive tasks and there's a lack of variety in what you do, this can lead to under-challenged burnout because you aren't being mentally stimulated. The typical trajectory of this type of burnout is that the tedium makes you feel cynical toward work, which leads to exhaustion and feeling detached, which leads to you becoming less effective—say, not bothering to prepare for things or forgetting to do things you've said you would. This detachment may be experienced as indifference toward things that you used to care about.

A parent or caregiver with high-need dependents repeating the cycle of preparing meals, cleaning up, and tending to personal care can feel monotony and intellectual understimulation, which means they aren't getting enough "healthy" stress to perform well. (We will look more at healthy versus unhealthy stress in Chapter 2.) But this can also happen in workplace settings, even when the work appears on the face of it to be intellectually stimulating. A veterinarian friend of mine who specialized in cardiology told me her daily cases had become so similar that she had taken on extra research projects to keep herself engaged and guard against the repetitive pattern of her day-to-day cases. High-achieving individuals can be at a greater risk of this type of burnout, since they tend to seek out challenges and thrive on being stretched.

Worn-Out Burnout
This isn't about the volume of work or how stimulating it is. Rather, it relates to how aligned your work is with your personal values or the sense of achievement you get from it. For example, if you work for a department that was originally set up to help people improve their mental health with therapy, but the targets only allow you to offer six sessions to a client and you know they'll need at least sixteen, this conflicts with your values and your ability to get a sense of achievement from the work. And it is exacerbated if your efforts aren't being acknowledged. The worn-out trajectory tends to start with emotional exhaustion and feeling low. Over a sustained period, this physically weighs you down, so you cope by trying to hold it all at arm's length, detaching to avoid caring as much. More experienced staff are more likely to associate with this subtype.

At the sharp end of this type of burnout is moral injury—a reaction to an acute episode of either witnessing things you disagree with or being expected to behave in ways that conflict with your morals. The effect is a shift in your foundational beliefs about yourself or the world, such as feelings of self-disgust or a loss of trust in others. Originally seen as an issue for military personnel, it was also observed in staff working in emergency and medical settings during the pandemic and adds to the reason why so many of these settings have found it hard.

ROLES THAT INCREASE VULNERABILITY TO BURNOUT

There are several roles in life that can contribute to us experiencing burnout because they create extra layers of stress, and I have broken these down as follows:

Parenting
Being a parent brings a lot of stress and monotony, the burden of this being highest when children are small and particularly

needy. Nevertheless, the challenges of parenthood continue as children develop, with new ones to navigate as they grow and become more independent. Parental burnout manifests within Maslach's three domains, where the telltale signs of emotional exhaustion are accompanied by a feeling of detachment from the child/children—for example, parents will often say things like, "I love my kids, but I can't stand to be around them." And then there is a constant sense of failure as a parent. Research into parental temperament suggests that those at higher risk of parental burnout and lacking skills in coping with strong emotions find it hard to switch tasks quickly and find stimulation, such as noise and demands, harder to process. Protective factors include having a strong identity as a parent—for example, if you always wanted to be a parent—and having support from family or a close-knit group of parent friends.

Caring for Others

In 2019, around 13 percent of adults over fifty provided informal care at least once a week for another adult, and with an aging population this will increase. The burden of caring, and therefore prolonged stress, increases the longer you care for someone, the more dependent they are on you and the poorer your relationship is with associated medical professionals. Buffers to informal-caregiver burnout include having strong social support and a positive relationship with the person you're caring for. Certain diseases where the dependent is abusive can put an extra strain on caregivers. Research in Poland that surveyed the needs of informal caregivers of dependents being cared for at home showed that the caregivers had *more* unmet needs than the people they were caring for, and that this increased the risk of burnout.

Studying

In cases of student burnout, there is a strong link between the number of demands, such as multiple deadlines and assessments, and lack of resources to cope, such as teacher support, pastoral care, stress-management techniques, and a peer group. Medical students have been a very well-researched group with rates of burnout ranging from 7.3 percent to 75.2 percent (depending on the country and measures of burnout used). The highly demanding nature of this course is considered to be responsible with regular assessments, practical assignments, and work placements in busy medical settings that are also stretched.

Poorly Managed Workplaces

Surveys from multiple employment sectors show how employee burnout is problematic in many professions, from corporate jobs to health and social care, engineers, lawyers, accountants, teachers, and police service. With a large formal organization around you there can be a lot of potential areas that could be adding to burnout in the way things are run, such as micromanagement, stringent targets, lack of autonomy, poor resource provision, and so on. Moreover, when policies and leadership fail to operate compassionately, their employees' needs aren't being well tended to. They get less job satisfaction and may struggle with work–life balance, and this leads to employee burnout. Burnout has been a big problem in the public sector, especially in caring professions, for a number of years now due to this.

Being a Leader

Leadership roles can be lonely and hold a lot of emotional demands, leaving leaders also vulnerable to burnout. Of course, burned-out leaders cannot provide high-quality management to their staff which has a knock-on impact. For example, they may make more demands of their team, put off making important decisions, and become impatient or less respectful of others' boundaries. All of this creates a toxic workplace culture—something that we will look at in more detail in Chapter 12.

Being Your Own Boss
The strains that entrepreneurs, freelancers, and sole traders face are slightly different than those of paid employees. They often shoulder the burden of uncertainty when starting a new venture, knowing that there is a risk involved to the survival of their company and any employees. They can be in a position of wearing multiple hats, especially in the early days, so have a lot to do and frequently report that this bleeds into their personal time. As in the case of leaders within established companies, theirs can be a lonely role with few appropriate people to seek emotional support from. A buffer to the burden of stress in entrepreneurial burnout is having autonomy, since entrepreneurs are in a position to make decisions about what they do, although they may not always have the resources or perhaps the courage to do so.

The good news is that for all these groups there is research showing that there can be positive buffers to their stress, including nervous-system management and social support. Improving your emotional intelligence—the ability to understand, be guided by, and manage your emotions—to manage stress is all part of this. Most importantly, these can be learned at any age, and we will be looking at how to go about this in Parts 3 and 4.

MENTAL- AND PHYSICAL-HEALTH DIAGNOSES WITH SIMILAR CHARACTERISTICS TO BURNOUT

Bear in mind that other factors could be contributing to how you're feeling. Untangling different mental-health and stress-related issues can be tricky, even for professionals, and it's also possible to have physical- or mental-health issues and conditions co-occurring with burnout compounding how you feel.

In the following chapters we will delve more into the human stress and trauma response and its cumulative effect on our bodies. There are numerous studies showing how our organs and bodily systems are compromised by overexposure to stress hormones without opportunities for proper rest and recuperation. Cardiovascular illness, diabetes, arthritis, chronic fatigue syndrome (CFS), and irritable bowel syndrome (IBS) are a few examples of physical ailments. What's more, unresolved burnout can lead to the body and brain trying to shut down or cope in a way that may meet other mental-health diagnostic criteria, too. In the case of Anika, who we met at the start of this chapter, the official diagnosis on her medical records was panic disorder, but this led her to me and we traced her issues back to soldiering on through the signs of burnout.

The health issues outlined here all have similar characteristics to burnout.

*Mental-Health Diagnoses**
These refer to the diagnostic categories of DSM-5:

NEURODIVERGENCE
While neurodivergence (such as ADHD and autism) doesn't cause the difficulties seen in burnout per se, it could be that masking your natural way of interacting with the world, to

---

*A quick note on mental-health diagnoses. A psychiatric diagnosis is a label that might be given to an individual whose behavior or emotional responses match a commonly observed pattern. They do not indicate that something invisible is going on below the surface to cause this. Such diagnoses therefore differ from *physical*-health diagnoses in which there are underlying biological causes, infection, or anatomical anomalies.

reduce feelings of being seen as different, has worn you down. Your masking behaviors may have become so habitual that you may not even be aware that's what you are doing anymore. Living in a world that prioritizes the needs of neurotypical people is hard work, so this could contribute to any exhaustion, cynicism, and low confidence you are experiencing. Assessments for this can be accessed via specialists and medical practitioners.

ANXIETY

Although the feeling of anxiety often occurs in burnout, anxiety diagnoses like obsessive compulsive disorder (OCD), health anxiety, and generalized anxiety disorder (GAD) are separate. The difference is usually in the nature, frequency, and intensity of intrusive thoughts (unpleasant thoughts that pop into your head uninvited), which may cluster around a theme. In health anxiety, intrusive thoughts will be focused on health worries; in OCD, they are likely to be fears about harm coming to someone close; and in GAD it is common to worry about things going wrong or not being able to cope (in addition, these worrisome thoughts lead to strong urges to take action to prevent bad things from happening; these urges are known as compulsions or safety behaviors).

DEPRESSION

You would meet a diagnosis of "clinical depression" if you presented with at least five of the following difficulties and they persisted for more than two weeks, troubling you for the majority of the day:

- Depressed mood
- A marked decline in interest in activities
- Cognitive difficulties affecting concentration, decision-making, and attention

- Beliefs of low self-worth
- Hopelessness about the future
- Recurrent thoughts of death
- Changed sleep (oversleeping or insomnia)
- Significant change in appetite (eating more or less)
- Psychomotor retardation (slowing down)
- Reduced energy and fatigue

Depression is an experience generally brought on by difficult life events and circumstances. Adverse situations like a lack of control over one's circumstances, having no one to turn to, oppression, inequality, uncertainty, and lack of close relationships can lead to feelings of hopelessness, very low self-worth, and the inability to find joy in anything. These adverse situations in depression are more broad-ranging than those typically associated with burnout. Researchers now generally agree that in the case of burnout we are looking at the impact of an acute, chronic stress response from prolonged imbalance around work.

Physical-Health Issues

The body and brain are not separate entities, so physical health can be negatively affected in burnout and, in fact, can often be the reason people are forced to slow down or seek help.

POST-VIRAL OR POST-INJURY

Recovery from physical-health conditions can take time, often longer than we realize, and can cause exhaustion and emotional stress, too.

CHRONIC FATIGUE SYNDROME

CFS is a complicated syndrome characterized by exhaustion, muscle aches, and brain fog. Typically, the fatigue from this comes in waves with good days and bad rather than feeling consistently exhausted as is more typical in burnout.

NUTRITIONAL DEFICIENCY

This can be assessed with a blood test to check your levels of minerals and vitamins. Iron, calcium, and vitamins C, D, and B12 are particularly important for energy and cognitive function.

HORMONE CHANGES—IN BOTH MEN AND WOMEN

Fluctuations in hormones impact our bodies physically. Research shows low testosterone in men can lead to fatigue, low mood, and insomnia.

The reasons for hormone changes vary and, indeed, stress is one possible cause. Women experience hormone fluctuations during perimenopause, typically in their forties, when the production of estrogen and progesterone gradually declines. A reduction in sex hormones has been shown to be a factor in brain fog, fatigue, mood changes, and difficulty sleeping, all closely aligned with difficulties seen in burnout. Determining whether the cause is burnout or menopause—or both—would involve checking for the nonoverlapping characteristics, such as the reduced sense of accomplishment from the work you are doing and emotional detachment that are common in burnout.

IS IT BURNOUT OR COULD THIS BE SOMETHING ELSE?

There are self-assessment tools for burnout available that you can easily access by searching online. Here are some of the options:

- Maslach Burnout Inventory (MBI) is the original workplace-burnout assessment that has been validated

---

and used in many studies. It separates the questions into the three domains of burnout difficulties to show you which areas you're struggling with the most. There are also variations specific to educators, medical personnel, human-services personnel, and students. The MBI is copyrighted and therefore available for a small fee. All these versions are available at www.MindGarden.com (an online psychological assessment website).

- If you'd like to access a free tool, the Copenhagen Burnout Inventory (CBI) is available easily online. This was developed following criticisms about the MBI (for example, that some people had negative reactions to the way questions were worded and that it wasn't culturally appropriate in some countries, such as Denmark, where the CBI originated).
- The Parental Burnout Assessment (PBA) is also available for free online; it has twenty-three questions about your feelings toward being a parent, exhaustion levels, and perception of coping with parenting.
- The Informal Caregiver Burnout Inventory (ICB-10) is a free, short ten-question assessment that measures burnout dimensions in addition to levels of social and professional support for caring duties (an important protective factor).

WHEN DO PEOPLE USUALLY REALIZE THEY'RE BURNED OUT?

Different people will eventually clock that they are burned out due to different circumstances. Here are some of the most common ones:

- **A Big Mistake:** When the exhaustion, disengagement, and brain fog (poor concentration and memory) affect your ability to function to the point that you make an error that cannot be ignored.

- **Physical "Crash":** When someone is off work, out sick, or admitted to hospital for a medical issue. In my therapy sessions with burnout individuals, I have seen this range from losing the ability to speak for short periods and having non-epileptic seizures to heart palpitations and feeling unable to get out of bed or suffering from intense panic attacks.

- **Too Many Unhealthy Coping Behaviors:** When someone is emotionally distressed or physically exhausted they will often default to the quickest distraction or pick-me-up possible. These behaviors can feel impulsive, and they often regret them afterward. Over time they find themselves living in a way that's very misaligned with their core values. This realization, or the strong sense of regret for behaving like this, can help people to see how burned out they are and lead them to finally seek help. Typical unhealthy coping behaviors that I'm referring to include eating junk food, impulsively shopping, ignoring messages from friends and family, drinking alcohol or using drugs, and losing chunks of time to scrolling social media.

- **Showing Up to Therapy for an Apparently Unrelated Problem:** This includes feeling floored by a setback at work or an argument with a friend and being concerned they haven't coped with an apparently small life event in their usual way. Often a relatively minor stressor becomes the straw that breaks the camel's back after months of slow-burning burnout in the background.

- **A Colleague or Family Member Calls It Out When They Notice Things Aren't Right:** Perhaps the burnout sufferer has dropped some balls, forgotten something super important, or is habitually sending emails at 2 a.m. A general deterioration in efficacy is another observable pattern often picked up by friends, family, and colleagues.

Often people only acknowledge their burnout once their day-to-day functioning has been affected to the point that it cannot be ignored; the elastic band isn't bouncing back into shape as it always used to. This can be scary and confusing, especially for someone whose identity up to that point included being the dependable one who gets things done no matter what. When we have big shifts in how we see ourselves, the world, or those around us, this feels traumatic.

THE FIVE STAGES OF BURNOUT

In the 1980s, associate professor for the School of Public Health and Nursing, Robert Veninga, along with urban anthropologist, Dr. James Spradley, developed a five-stage model* depicting how job satisfaction degrades into disillusionment followed by physical and mental difficulties that overwhelm the individual. This has now become a frequently referenced model of how stress progresses into clinical burnout.

Stage 1: Honeymoon
At this stage, you feel generally satisfied with what you're doing and achieving, and your energy levels for your projects are good. You may be driven and enthusiastic about what you're doing but struggle to pace yourself. Even though this isn't the stage when you'll notice any distress that feels like burnout, being able to recognize it allows you to take steps to prevent yourself from progressing to the next stage.

---

*Stage models can oversimplify issues and suggest a linear trajectory. This is particularly relevant in the case of burnout because it isn't a uniform experience. However, all aspects of burnout include an element of elevated stress, which this most commonly used five-stage model is helpful for depicting.

Signs you might be here:

- Saying "yes" to the projects you're engaged in feels exciting and easy.
- You are led by your enthusiasm or drive for positive outcomes rather than practicalities.
- You don't feel like tending to other life duties, hobbies, or social connections as much as usual.
- Boundaries between work and personal life feel blurred because of your passion and excitement.

Stage 2: Onset of Stress

The projects lose their shine as the reality of the demands takes over. Typical external pressures that are important to highlight at this stage are: having too much to do, being deprived of agency, feeling criticized that your efforts aren't rewarded or that you are being treated unfairly, and feeling socially unsupported. Without any buffers to stress in place, your body reacts with its stress response, meaning that physiological changes happen inside you (more on these in Chapter 2). People who proceed to the next stage tend to overlook how stressed they are starting to feel at this point.

Signs you might be here:

- You get irritable or impatient around minor issues (being asked a favor, people walking slowly, or someone telling a long-winded story).
- Your brain starts to race, and worries are hard to dismiss.
- You are questioning whether you've taken on too much, but at the same time you now feel committed.
- You find it hard to switch off; you want to rest or sleep but find it challenging to do so.

- You neglect your personal needs.
- If you take a moment to tune in to your body (which you probably aren't doing very much), you'll notice tension and a sense of urgency to rush and make quick decisions.

Stage 3: Chronic Stress

If your initial stress isn't addressed, the longer-lasting physical impacts of stress start to take effect. You might start to notice the physical toll of this but are likely in denial about how stressed you're feeling.

Signs you might be here—you match a lot of the signs in Stage 2 and in addition:

- You overreact to things quickly with anxiety, annoyance, or low mood.
- You have stressed emotional reactions like panic attacks, bouts of irritability, or paralysis.
- You have physical stress signs, such as headaches, back pain, catching colds easily, or reduced libido.
- You have cognitive signs of stress, such as difficulty making decisions, focusing, and concentrating.
- You have withdrawn from your social circles and hobbies.
- You are coping with stress in ways you don't feel good about, such as emotional eating, doomscrolling, drinking more, procrastinating, seeking reassurance, or impulsive online shopping.
- Difficulty in resting might be causing insomnia or early morning waking.
- You find it hard to admit to yourself that you are feeling as stressed as you are.

Stage 4: Burnout

Now you've reached burnout. At first, you may not be aware you are here, because you continue to function despite starting to feel wrung out. You become avoidant of making decisions but when you do manage to make them they are less rational (this includes decisions around self-care to stop progression to the next stage of burnout). You are also more likely to compare yourself unfavorably to others; where previously you may have felt inspired by others you look up to, now you feel less confident about your own abilities and are more likely to identify with those who actually aren't as capable as you.

Signs you might be here—you match a lot of the points from Stage 3 and in addition:

- You feel physically depleted.
- You get bouts of apathy or indifference toward your work or events that previously lit you up.
- You feel cynical or resentful toward others, your work, or the prospect of change being possible.
- You feel helpless or self-critical about your ability to achieve good outcomes.
- You get bouts of feeling detached from what's going on around you like you're only half present, struggling to connect with others and with your activities.
- You have brain fog which causes you to make mistakes, such as missing appointments, forgetting to reply to emails, ordering the wrong item from the internet, etc.
- You feel low in mood and trapped here; you get thoughts of escapism—for example, something happening that would mean you can finally have a break, like getting ill or injuring yourself, so no one expects anything from you.

- Transition points in the day are tricky—either rushing between them and finding it hard to switch gear for what is required of you next or finding it hard to initiate the next activity (like getting out of the shower or cleaning up after dinner).
- You may have noticed changes in your weight—either a loss from lack of appetite or gain from the effects of cortisol and poor self-care.
- You feel alone with all of this.

Stage 5: Habitual Burnout

Burnout patterns set in further and become severe. More of the signs of distress (see page 21) are resonating with you, and you are suffering them more intensely. Your body shifts up a gear from sending the "quieter" messages that it was reaching its limits during previous stages (aches and pains) to full-on "shouting" at you to stop and slow down (palpitations, zoning out, or becoming numb or depressed). The elastic band has lost its shape and bounce completely, or it might feel more accurate to describe it as having snapped.

Signs you might be here—all the signs of Stages 2, 3, and 4 and in addition:

- Your day-to-day functioning isn't what it was, and others may now have noticed the change in your mood and cognitive functioning or that you keep "dropping balls."
- The physical signs of stress are now impossible to ignore, such as aches and pains, palpitations, zoning out, panic attacks, or finding it hard to speak.
- Not only do you keep catching colds but you take longer to recover from each one.
- The brain fog might be more intense, such as forgetting key things and great difficulty in concentrating.

- Depression and feeling hopeless about feeling better or how to come back from this; this could include suicidal thoughts, too.

It's helpful to think of burnout as a continuum rather than as an "I-either-have-it-or-I-don't" concept. At one end of the continuum are the milder difficulties that may not fully feature on someone's radar. The middle section is where stress starts to cause problems. Then at the severe end lies clinical burnout where the impact on your physical, mental, and emotional functioning is such that you cannot carry out your usual day-to-day tasks.

In Stage 5, it's likely that something has interrupted the cycle of busyness and work and enforced a stop, perhaps with the help of a therapist or intervention at work or a period of sick leave. Recovery from this stage takes time, though—an average of one to three years for someone to return to work and feel like they were functioning at full capacity if it's severe, according to the research. So it's important to have realistic expectations about how long it takes for your nervous system to recalibrate. Progress is slow and steady.

The people who psychologists like myself are also concerned about are those who sit for long periods at the mid to lower end of the continuum (Stages 2–4). They appear to function well but are likely masking emotional and physical exhaustion. Their friends, family, and colleagues probably haven't noticed, and they themselves don't realize this level of stress is not OK.

Being anywhere on the burnout continuum if it is left unaddressed is bad for both your quality of life and long-term health. Wishful thoughts about escaping life's stresses or a hopelessness about being able to change your situation are signs that something needs to change. You should listen to them, but all too often people don't...

WHY DO WE IGNORE THE SIGNS OF STRESS?

There are many pressures that make it hard for us to listen to the cues of stress in our bodies and take appropriate action, and they can be broadly divided into two types: external and internal.

External Pressures: From the People or Situations Around Us

This includes any demands in our lives, such as bills to pay, quarterly targets, a high case load, or children with never-ending questions and wants. Often these external pressures can creep up so slowly that we either fail to spot the cumulative load or we feel unable to challenge them because each issue on its own seems small and inconsequential. For example, when I worked as a National Health Service (NHS) therapist, the creep looked something like this: we would be asked to fill in a new form for recording missed sessions; then asked to update a second database with outcome results; then told we had to start doing our own duties, like printing, sending letters, and so on. Over six years in the same department the administration for my clinics roughly doubled.

Specific external pressures in our work environments include:

- time pressures, such as deadlines (like completing projects or getting kids to their activities)
- conflicts or disagreements with others in your team or family
- high emotional labor—needing to tend to others' negative emotions which can be contagious without the right emotional support for ourselves
- work overload (too much to do)
- role ambiguity (being unsure what we should be doing and not wanting to step on the toes of others)
- lack of control of our situation, resources, or demands being made
- excessive criticism from people around us

- lack of positive feedback or appreciation
- job insecurity
- too many complex tasks
- financial worries

Within workplace settings, occupational psychologists often get involved in finding solutions to address these external pressures. This is important because you so often cannot do this alone. However, some external pressures are less visible as they come from cultural ideals about our roles and what's expected of us— for example, women as caregivers or men as breadwinners. These lead others to treat us in a certain way or make stereotyped demands of us that are hard to push back from. They also contribute to negative beliefs about ourselves and our ability to cope with it all (more on this in Chapter 7).

Internal Pressures: Pressures Inside Us, Like Emotions or Thoughts
These include anything that arises *inside* of us, motivating us to keep going despite our stress. This is informed by our biological and psychological makeup, such as personality traits, core beliefs, or sensitivity to stimuli and temperament. It shows up as:

- emotions like guilt, anxiety, and shame
- thoughts like "I'm responsible for keeping things together" or "I've not done enough to deserve a break yet"
- unpleasant sensations in the body, such as a rush of adrenaline that makes everything feel urgent, tenses muscles, races the heart, or causes bouts of fidgetiness

Neuroticism is a personality trait that consistently correlates highly with burnout. Someone scoring high on neuroticism has a tendency to worry and to experience stronger and more frequent negative emotions than someone with a low score. That is to say: these people experience intense internal pressures.

There are three patterns of internal pressures I regularly see when working in therapy with people who feel burned out.

- **Perfectionism:** trying to get things "just so" at the expense of your well-being
- **People-Pleasing:** taking on too much responsibility for the well-being of others, again at your own expense
- **Avoidance of Negative Emotions:** a belief that you need to avoid negative feelings because you don't feel equipped to cope with them, using busyness and work to do so

The fictious case studies in this book (Anika, Scott, Suraj, and Sarah) all fit with at least one of these, although they are not stand-alone problems and can co-occur. Part 2 of this book will help to map out the reasons why these internal pressures develop to be so strong, while Part 3 will provide ways to overcome them.

HOW TO SPOT BURNOUT WHEN YOU ARE IN THE THICK OF IT

It's hard to spot burnout when you are at the lower end of the continuum or before it becomes clinical and you stop functioning. What's more, the people around you will be benefiting from your overworking behaviors because you're getting a lot of stuff done, so while they are not necessarily deliberately manipulating you, they may not be motivated to pause and reflect on the unhealthy nature of some of your behaviors or be equipped to help you see this yourself.

Scott's Wednesday Evening: An Example of Someone in Stage 4 of Burnout

Scott stopped for milk on the way home. His daughter's tennis practice had overrun, so it was getting late, and yet he didn't think twice about swiping open a work email when his phone buzzed. His daughter rolled her eyes from the back seat. How come he was always telling her to put her phone down but always glued to his!

"Congratulations on your new venue," read the message. This was the email he'd been anticipating for months as he worked tirelessly toward this outcome. Late nights writing proposals, anxious planning of staff and moving funds, constant checking that he hadn't missed anything...And now it had all paid off. This email confirmed: He had done it!

However, he felt no elation or burst of pride. Instead, he slipped his phone back into his pocket and started the engine. The to-do list in his head had just exploded with all the new things he would now need to jump on tomorrow. No, it would need to be tonight if he wanted it done right. He was exhausted, but he'd push through. He wouldn't be able to sleep anyway because he would think about what needed to be done. And now he had the new worry that this new venue would mean he had bitten off more than he could chew and maybe he wasn't cut out for this after all.

Driving home on autopilot, he slowly became aware that his daughter was talking to him. It took a moment to refocus on what she was saying—something about the tennis practice? He struggled to make sense of it. Oh, she was worried about the match on Saturday. He had a sense that he should do some "dad talk," but he couldn't seem to dredge up any words of comfort or to really connect with her concerns. He was sure she'd be fine.

His daughter waited for words of reassurance but realized her dad had slipped off into his own head again. She saw his shoulders were slumped. He looked tired. She wondered what he'd read on his phone to make him like this. Must have been bad news. She knew to leave him alone when he was like this or he'd just get annoyed.

Scott's behaviors reflect Maslach's three dimensions:

Physical and Emotional Exhaustion
Scott's daughter senses from his body language that he is tired and, although Scott experiences a few fleeting moments of heaviness at the prospect of his to-do list, he has grown too disconnected from his body to interpret the signs of fatigue fully in this moment.

Detachment
Scott seems uninterested in his daughter's issues. This is the empathy-distress fatigue in action. Scott also finds it hard to connect with what he is doing in the present moment (driving home from tennis with his daughter), and is disengaged from activities that feel good and from the people around him. He might be *physically* present, but his head is elsewhere, so he is struggling to listen or take things in.

Reduced Feeling of Personal Accomplishment
Scott just had a big "win" worthy of celebrating and shouting about but this doesn't even feature on his radar. He is so exhausted and overworked that he just shrugs and carries on, unable to appreciate what an achievement this is. Moreover, his fears that he isn't up for the job are very typical in burnout; even with evidence to the contrary—like Scott's flourishing business—there can be doubts.

When your behavior is frenetic, you have no mental space to consider how you feel or realize how disconnected you are from the people in your life. What started as a project Scott was passionate about at some point along the way became more demanding. Because this is often a creeping process, the level of stress can be tricky to pin down and quantify. We don't wake up one morning to find ourselves in burnout—it is a gradual experience which is another reason why it's so hard to spot.

So the demands being thrown at us come with a level of stress. If this gets too high and isn't addressed, it can begin to seem normal. When I have posted on social media about the signs of stress, comments like "you're just describing being a mom" or "that's just modern life" are testament to this. We've normalized excessive stress so much that we can no longer see it. There is also an undertone of anger to these comments, perhaps hinting at that trapped feeling or learned helplessness (see page 55). The sentiment is: "I have too much to do and I'm stressed, but I have to suck this up because I'm a mom, entrepreneur, academic, or doctor, and there's nothing anyone can do about it."

This sentiment is damaging. Chronic stress is toxic and can lead us into burnout. But how does this happen? At what point does stress stop being "just" stress and tip into something much harder to bounce back from?

Chapter 2

HOW CHRONIC STRESS LEADS TO BURNOUT

Before Anika was out sick with burnout, her stress had been bubbling under the surface for quite some time. When friends asked how she was, she rolled out her stock response—"I'm fine"—and her carefully applied makeup masked the scale of stress and anxiety beneath. The reality was that she couldn't tell if she was fine or not. She had spent months crashing from one demand to the next every day, carried by a nervous energy that eventually culminated in full-blown panic attacks.

Anika had progressed from Stage 1 of the burnout honeymoon phase in her newly promoted position into Stages 2 and 3 of the increased stress without realizing it. She had been caught here for a while with the stress leading to headaches, mild stomach problems, and aches in her back that she had not addressed, telling herself they weren't a big deal. If she had been attuned to this, she would have realized that it was an unhealthy level of stress and that she was operating almost permanently from a specific part of her autonomic nervous system called the sympathetic nervous system. This is not how humans were designed to live and operate in the long-term, though.

Your autonomic nervous system is your body's command center, transmitting messages from the brain to the body and vice versa. It enables you to respond appropriately to people and situations around you without the need for your conscious brain processes to get involved. It is therefore essential for survival, initiating responses to demands and threats with great speed when it perceives signs of trouble.

THE VAGAL NERVE—KEY TO CALM AND PRODUCTIVITY

An essential part of this messaging service is carried out by the vagal nerve: a bundle of fibers connecting the brain stem to most of the body's organs like the heart and gut, as well as peripheral parts like the facial muscles, ears, and neck. The vagal nerve is responsible for our responses to stress. It is constantly communicating via the brain stem any cues of safety or danger being picked up by the body. If your heart quickens at an unexpected bang in the street, you experience a flash of fear and a thought that tries to make sense of this, such as, "Is something bad happening?" This is your interoception at work—your ability to feel and listen to sensations in the body.

Eighty percent of the messages between brain and body travel from the body to the brain. When the body is calm, the brain perceives there to be no threat. This highlights both how helpful it is to understand what is happening at the physiological level and also why targeting the body's feeling of safety is so vital to feeling better from burnout.

We feel different emotions, behaviors, thoughts, and body reactions, depending on which branch of the nervous system is in control at any time. You could think of these as gears on a vehicle; I will refer to them as modes. In green mode we are mid-gear, going about the day with the sense that we are on top of things, not rushed, just generally content and engaged. Minor challenges like burnt toast and traffic jams are experienced simply as mild inconveniences from which we quickly bounce back.

In amber mode, the increased demands placed on us have switched us up a gear. This creates a sense of urgency and energy in the brain and body that prepares us for action. In this mode, our tolerance for the burnt toast and traffic jams is lower; not only do we get more agitated by these annoyances but the agitation endures for longer. We can accommodate a considerable level of stress in amber mode; however, we are not designed to remain in one high gear for too long as we will discover in this chapter.

Our red operating mode is a state of energy conservation and shutdown; our gear is now dropping into neutral. We can dip in and out of this for short periods without experiencing long-term problems. In fact, this allows deep rest which is good for us, as we will explore in the next chapter.

Like an automatic car, our autonomic nervous system should shift smoothly between modes depending on what is required. We cannot drive anywhere in one gear alone, so each part of our nervous system has a vital role and none of them should be demonized. But burnout can be the experience of getting stuck in amber or red (or oscillating between the two), unable to transition up and down the gears as required for the different people and situations in our day.

The good news is that a nervous system that has become stuck *can* recover, although this is a process that takes time and gentle persistence. We cannot recalibrate in just a few days.

Green Mode

Ideally, we should be spending most of our time here in green mode, because the organs involved in the general well-being of the body are then able to function at full capacity. We can digest food properly, accurately interpret body language or facial expressions, and feel safe enough to "switch off" when falling asleep or resting.

This relaxed state is made possible by the ventral vagal circuit—a branch of our parasympathetic nervous system that is active when we are not under threat (this is the most recent part of our nervous system to develop—recent being 200 million years ago). Its development allowed humans the freedom to explore and be curious and open to change. Most importantly, it allowed us to create the social connections essential to our survival because we thrive best in small communities. This is referred to as the social engagement system (more on this in Chapter 4), and it is linked with the release of the hormone called oxytocin which makes us feel calm and content.

When our systems want to come back to this calmer green mode for connection and rest, it can engage the vagal brake. This brake slows our heart rate which communicates to our other body systems that any danger has passed. Certain activities can promote this braking mechanism by pleasantly stimulating areas of the body where the ventral vagal nerve is clustered, such as slow breathing, yoga, singing, humming, laughing, and listening to or playing music. (I will give you tools for engaging your vagal brake in Chapter 5.)

Green mode, as well as affording us the more calm emotions, is a state that enables us to think clearly and rationally with our functional Intelligence Quotient (IQ) at maximum capacity, because the parts of the brain most engaged during green mode are the frontal lobes where our high-level, intelligent thinking processes are believed to be housed. Green mode is therefore the ideal mode for:

- **Problem-Solving:** Figuring out potential solutions and the logical steps to implement them.

- **Language:** Understanding what others are saying and being able to communicate back effectively.
- **Concentration and Attention:** Sustaining focus on a task.
- **Imagining the Future:** Seeing past the present moment and accessing strategies to improve your current situation (like what you need to do to reduce external stressors).
- **Creative Thought:** Linking dots and generating new ideas.
- **Memory for Events:** Remembering sequence and details.
- **Open and Rational Communication:** Allowing us to have connections to people around us.

When we switch out of green mode into amber mode, access to the frontal lobes reduces, which can make it hard to engage in certain activities that involve this part of the brain. Unfortunately, this can include activities that might be helpful for coping with task overload, such as journaling, time-management planning, and problem-solving. In fact, trying to implement these when you don't have enough of the green mode activated can end up adding to your experience of stress rather than reducing it, as you get frustrated with yourself for "failing" and start self-attacking (e.g., "others find journaling so easy but I don't even know where to start").

Amber Mode
Amber mode encompasses the automatic response in our bodies, emotions, and behaviors that kicks in when life gets demanding. When the messages from the nervous system signify that more energy and action are required to deal with all these demands, the vagal brake is released so that our hearts speed up. The body reactions we experience at this point are those we need to mobilize ourselves to take action in response to perceived threats. In modern life these threats might be a traffic jam or an angry email from the boss.

In amber mode, the sympathetic nervous system takes charge. It is much older than the ventral vagal branch of the parasympathetic nervous system, the branch that gives us green mode. It was created 400 million years ago and developed to respond to the evolving demands faced by our ancestors at the time, like the threat of predators, the possibility of being ostracized from the tribe, and long, hard winters when food was scarce. Amber mode motivated us to carry out activities to stay safe, for example by maintaining our social connections for support and gathering enough food for the winter. Contrary to popular belief, it isn't designed solely to respond to immediate threats; it also helps us to meet longer-term demands. We tap into this when we play; it's that energy we get when we do things for pleasure or when we are working on challenges and goals, like a promotion or personal-best time on a run. During these activities, our sympathetic nervous system lights up in a positive way known as eustress, giving us a pleasant buzz from the hormone dopamine and making us feel driven. Because this feels so good, we are inspired to seek out more of it, sometimes in quite an addictive way and at the expense of rest time in green mode. For example, when I gave a talk about stress management at a veterinary emergency department, the staff shared how confusing it was that, although they wished to feel less stressed, they preferred the days when there were multiple emergencies to tend to and they were running around compared to the slower clinics when they had less to do. This is because our nervous systems pump us with enough of the positive hormones like dopamine to keep us going. This makes for a "noisier" and more exciting experience than the gentler one we get from oxytocin in green mode, which is why we can so easily end up prioritizing activities that stimulate amber more. We therefore need to create the right context to allow ourselves to slow down into green, and so I worked with the veterinary team to think of ways for them to do this at work with a soothing station and check-ins with each other and gentler activities to focus on during quieter clinics. I will come back to ways in which we can create these calming contexts in Chapter 11.

A STATE OF FLOW

We *can* be in our alert amber mode without this being experienced as anxiety or unpleasant stress. This is where feelings of excitement and passion come from, which means, as we touched on earlier, stress is healthy for us *up to a point*, as demonstrated by the Yerkes–Dodson Law stress curve:

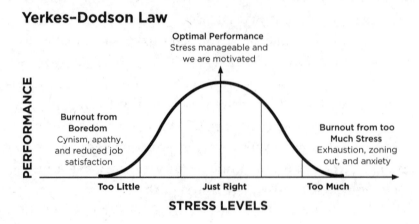

Yerkes–Dodson Law

Optimal Performance
Stress manageable and
we are motivated

PERFORMANCE

Burnout from
Boredom
Cynism, apathy,
and reduced job
satisfaction

Burnout from too
Much Stress
Exhaustion, zoning
out, and anxiety

Too Little   Just Right   Too Much

STRESS LEVELS

"If you want something done, ask a busy person" is a common expression that is supported by this stress curve: Our motivation and output peak when we are in the nonthreatening, energized amber mode. But if the stress mounts too high, the negative effects of the stress start to outweigh the positive, leading to the frenetic and worn-out patterns of burnout outlined in Chapter 1.

Interestingly, being in a state of "flow"—the rewarding experience of sustained, deep concentration in an activity—sits at the apex of this curve. You can get into flow with anything that you find interesting and pleasantly challenging, such as playing an instrument, gaming, reading, writing, and so on.

There are mixed findings about the state of flow and burnout, but typically the positive experience of flow provides a buffer to the negative effects of stress because the activity is enjoyable, aligned with your values, and stimulating. However, this state can be *so* positive that it becomes moreish and even addictive, leading people to neglect other areas of their lives— like relationships, hobbies, and rest time—as a result, to the point that these all deteriorate. For example, a partner who never gets to spend time with you may end the relationship. This leaves you vulnerable to burnout because when the stress mounts beyond your flow's comfort zone, you have no buffers left.

And what of the underchallenged pattern of burnout? How does this fit with the stress curve? Well, it is linked to boredom which sits at the start of this stress curve. Boredom has been shown to be highly aversive to humans. In one experiment carried out by professor of psychology at University of Virginia, Timothy Wilson, and colleagues in 2014, researchers asked participants to spend fifteen minutes alone in an undecorated room doing nothing with the option of pressing a button that would give them an electric shock. Results showed that 67 percent of men and 25 percent of women preferred an electric shock over doing nothing. This demonstrates our strong desire to be occupied in a stimulating way. It also helps us to understand how we tend to miss out on the opportunities to deeply rest because we find it so hard to tolerate a slower pace. The feelings of boredom that arise when we are resting motivate us to find stimulation again.

PROTECTION MODE

When the sympathetic nervous system reacts to protect us, we have an acute stress response. Our body scans and perceives threat before we are consciously aware, a process referred to as neuroception. These are threats from both our physical surroundings and inside our bodies, akin to an internal smoke alarm always scanning in the background for signs of smoke. The body signals include even subtle changes within our organs, such as gut or heart rate, that we may not be consciously aware of.

At the point when a threat is perceived, the adrenal glands release the stress hormones cortisol and adrenaline, and each organ in the body receives a shot of these, immediately shifting things up a gear so we can move fast. Our hearts race to get the blood to the large muscle groups, ready to run or fight, our breathing becomes rapid to oxygenate all the blood effectively, and the blood is diverted from nonessential functioning (like the digestion of food) to give extra support to the parts of the body involved in survival. These physiological changes of the organs into survival mode are called *allostatic responses.*

At the same time, changes take place in the brain: Blood flow shifts from the frontal lobes to the threat-response center (the amygdala). This causes our focus of attention to narrow and our thoughts to become threat-focused, leading to "what if" worries and catastrophizing (imagining the worst-case scenario), all of which allows us to preempt and prepare for potential problems. The other reaction in amber mode is anger which creates in us an urge to defend ourselves. Anger can look like full-blown rage, but it will show up more often in the socially acceptable forms of frustration and irritation. We refer to these as our "fight-or-flight" responses.

The body's acute stress response was designed to activate us to get to safety quickly (escape the predator) and then to discharge any excess adrenaline and oxygen that are no longer needed so we return to our green mode quickly. This discharge process is supported by movement or shaking of the muscles. This brings the protective stress response to an end at which point our other important bodily functions can resume—like digestion, the ability to rest, and reengagement with our social group that enables us to maintain our safety net.

POSITIVE STRESS

There are helpful internal consequences of a short burst of stress like this, all designed to get us through the moment as effectively as possible:

- **Enhanced Immunity:** As the body prepares for the possibility of injury, any wounds will heal quickly and stay protected from infection.
- **Sharper Cognitive Abilities:** Due to the production of neurotrophins—proteins that support brain neurons which allow a narrowing of concentration—we can focus on the task in hand.
- **Surge in Motivation:** This helps get the job done.
- **Improved Physical Strength:** Our muscles get a surge of adrenaline (particularly helpful for athletes).

FIVE WAYS THAT MODERN LIFE KEEPS YOU IN AMBER MODE

1. Modern life is extremely stimulating of our senses in a way that we haven't yet adapted to. This means that even if we aren't in protection mode, our sympathetic nervous system may be "on" anyway due to bombardment from noisy shopping malls, screen overload, and excessive choice in the form of well-being apps, TV shows, and so on.

---

2. Technology makes it hard to step out of "doing" and "achieving." Many people multitask when supposedly resting, such as doing their online food shopping while watching TV, replying to texts while waiting for their coffee to brew, and so on. Again, these may seem like innocuous activities, but they prevent any nervous system reset from happening.

3. We don't get enough opportunities to engage in activities that help us to discharge the stress hormones so we can return to baseline. These include physical exercise, play, connecting with others (talking and laughing), rhythmic breathing, and creative activity.

4. Because of the level of choice and the ability to act on impulses, we tend to rush from one activity to another. These demands rarely stop, meaning that our sympathetic nervous system remains online all the time, interfering with our other essential "green mode" functions— cue sleep difficulties, digestive issues, and feeling socially isolated or lonely.

5. Fear of missing out (FOMO) comes from the threat response being activated when we see our social group doing something without us. Our threat centers fear being cast out of the tribe, which for our ancestors would have spelled death. Unfortunately, nowadays, we have social media telling us all the (supposedly) amazing things others are doing, so my clients often report feeling FOMO, which leads them to say "yes" to more social events. We can't help it.

TOXIC STRESS

Chronic stress isn't just a longer-lasting version of short-term stress. There are physical and psychological changes that happen if stress hormones are released for too long.

When our allostatic responses (the changes made by our bodily systems to respond to the threats) remain "on," it causes a build-up referred to as the allostatic load. Not only does this lead to system wear and tear, but without the recovery time it leads to the systems growing weary or overly sensitive. This can cause lethargy, dulled reactions (like zoning out), and reduced emotional repertoire (like not caring)—all common complaints in burnout.

During amber mode the body burns through energy quickly, so when this is depleted it will demand quick replenishment for its reserves. So now the cravings for high-carb foods kick in, since this is the fastest way for the body to access more calories. If this type of snacking continues for too long, especially if there is also a lack of nutrients coming in from well-balanced meals, then the body doesn't have the essential building blocks it needs to recover from the wear and tear. All of this starts to take its toll on us.

How Toxic Stress Takes Its Toll
  * **On Our Brains:** Our ability to grow new brain cells is essential to maintain our cognitive abilities throughout our lifetimes, but this growth of new brain cells is interrupted when there is an excess of stress hormones. The interruption affects the areas in the frontal lobes associated with executive functioning: emotion regulation, language, appropriate management of our behaviors, memory, and our ability to visualize. All of this has a knock-on effect on our ability to make reasoned decisions and plan.

    The other part of our brain affected by toxic stress is the threat-response region, the amygdala, which becomes more sensitive. This means we are more likely to misinterpret any ambiguous information as dangerous, and our concentration can be scattered as our brains can't work out where to focus. Everything seems to be an emergency and we get the urge to rush. This contributes to brain fog, difficulties staying on task, and problems remembering things. Our functional IQ can drop up to twenty points as a result of all of this.

- **On Our Bodies:** Whereas in short-term stress immunity is temporarily improved to help us fight off infection in a moment of crisis, high allostatic load causes it to drop due to wear and tear on the organs and causes excess cortisol, resulting in inflammation, which is why we become more susceptible to bugs and viruses at this point.

  Wounds take longer to heal, and we are not only more susceptible to disease and illness, but it takes us longer to get better. Headaches and joint pains are the most common physical experiences associated with burnout, particularly in the large muscle groups, such as the back and shoulders where we tend to hold tension. We may also experience problems with the gut like IBS. This is the digestive system in amber mode responding to the stress by diverting blood away from the gut toward larger muscle groups, like our arms and legs, ready to run or fight. Over time, this results in a lower absorption of nutrients because the digestive system isn't carrying out its business as usual.

  Finally, and sadly sometimes fatally, there is the impact on the cardiovascular system with an increase in blood pressure and heart rate. This may not be observable in the short-term but can contribute to conditions like stroke and heart attacks in the long-term.

- **On Our Sleep:** Sleep comes easily when we feel safe (i.e., in green mode), but our ancestors may have gambled with their lives if they had been able to fall into an unconscious state of sleep for seven to eight hours during times of threat. This is why our systems are not wired to switch off when our stress is high and why so many people with chronic stress struggle with falling or staying asleep or only manage low-quality slumber; they can only achieve light sleep.

Without decent rest, the body's ability to restore itself declines. The cleansing of toxins from brain and body that usually happens in deep sleep cannot be carried out, and the process that reduces the emotional charge from our memories during dream sleep fails to take place, and so we carry these emotional experiences into the next day without the fresh perspective that a dream sleep would bring.

We all know how exhausted, grumpy, and overwhelmed we feel after just one night of poor sleep. If all the restorative sleep functions keep being missed, it means our reserves keep on being depleted. Over time, this further impacts on our ability to focus and make decisions.

- **On Our Emotions:** Emotions communicate our needs in any given situation. They come hardwired with behavior patterns to help us stay safe. We have a large repertoire of emotions that we will look at in Chapter 10. When we are in amber mode, the full range is reduced, and the emotions available to us are: anger (ranging from mild frustration or agitation to rage) and anxiety (ranging from a sense of anticipation to panic). Sadness and joy are green-mode emotions. We can feel them only when we feel safe enough. They enable us to show the compassion and empathy essential for human connection. They also enable us to feel compassion for ourselves and allow us to let others in to support us.

Over time, with limited access to other emotions and with overrepresented anger and/or anxiety, we experience emotional fatigue—feelings of helplessness and inadequacy. This explains why some people in burnout become very cynical or seem to be giving up.

- **On Our Behaviors:** Finally, this negative load on our brains, bodies, sleep, and emotions can lead to behaviors designed for a quick fix. This is when our good intentions and routines around eating well, getting enough sleep, and exercise may dissolve. We reach for the quick energy boost in the form of convenience food, the quick dopamine hit in the form of scrolling the web, or the quick sedative effects that alcohol brings.

USING ALCOHOL TO UNWIND AT THE END OF THE DAY

Why do we so often turn to a beer or a glass of wine at the end of a long day? It's helpful to understand why we find alcohol so appealing during periods of toxic stress.

A key effect of alcohol is that it enhances gamma-aminobutyric acid (GABA), a neurotransmitter responsible for inhibiting our responses. Or to put it another way, GABA slows down our thoughts and reactions. When thoughts are racing at 100 miles an hour, this calming effect is exactly what we crave, so it's no wonder that we reach for the quickest (and often socially accepted) way of achieving it.

So if alcohol relaxes us and has a sedative effect, why shouldn't we use it to help with burnout issues like falling asleep and difficulty relaxing? Well, with time, we develop a tolerance for the sedative effects of alcohol and start to require more of it to achieve the same calming results. A comprehensive review of sleep studies was carried out in 2016 by psychiatry professor Gustavo Angarita and his team into insomnia and the use of alcohol (and other substances). They found that heavy alcohol consumption generally makes it harder to fall asleep and reduces the total time sleeping and the duration of deep (restorative) stages of sleep achieved (including REM sleep).

If this has developed into a bigger problem for you already, you may need professional support to detox and recover. If you are reading this and realizing that the bottle of wine in the fridge is emptying faster than it used to but you don't think you are dependent on it, then now is the time to take some proactive steps to improve this.

Try:

- putting all your alcohol away (in the shed or a locked cupboard) out of view so it's harder to reach for
- buying alcohol-free alternatives
- looking at Chapter 14 of this book for alternative wind down routines for sleep

VICIOUS CYCLE

All these negative impacts on the body, mind, sleep, and emotions are self-perpetuating and create a vicious cycle, trapping us in burnout.

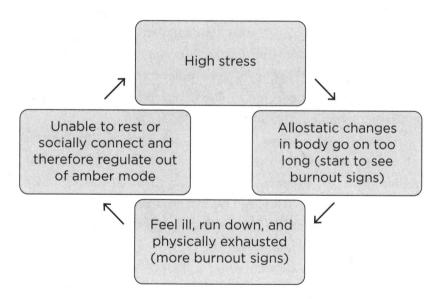

This vicious cycle can only go on for so long, until your nervous system tips into another place: the trauma response.

HOW PROLONGED CHRONIC STRESS
TRIGGERS A TRAUMA RESPONSE

Trauma is not the same as post-traumatic stress disorder (PTSD). PTSD is a mental-health diagnosis given when someone presents with specific complaints, like a heightened startle reflex, along with scary experiences called "trauma-reliving" (nightmares or flashbacks). For a PTSD diagnosis, an individual will usually have been involved in or witnessed a terrifying event.

The term "trauma" refers to a broader range of experiences, and trauma-trained therapists tend to differentiate between the type of trigger event involved in PTSD: big-T trauma and little-t trauma. Some examples of little-t traumas I have seen in my practice include being rejected by someone who matters to the trauma sufferer and being humiliated or bullied—perhaps by a teacher or mentor, a parent, or a peer at school.

Renowned Canadian physician and author Gabor Maté defines trauma not as what happens *to* you but as "what happens *inside you* as a result of what happened to you." Even little-t traumas can result in long-lasting nervous-system responses, particularly when there is an accumulation of similar little-ts, such as being repeatedly ignored or criticized, setting unrealistic goals, being bullied, and so on.

In the case of burnout, little-ts from your early life feed the internal pressures I refer to in Chapter 1, such as perfectionism, people-pleasing, or using busyness to distract yourself from negative emotions. Although you may have developed these behaviors in response to events that were humiliating or made you feel rejected, originally for the purpose of protecting your-self, they may now be doing you a disservice. People-pleasing may be the internal pressure that stops you delegating. Perfection and using busyness as a distraction may be what are constantly driving you beyond your limits and into burnout.

However, little-ts don't occur only in early life. They can also accumulate in adult life and contribute to burnout, such as the trainee doctor humiliated by her consultant in front of her peers, the phone constantly ringing with emergencies when you're "on call" at home, the incessant emails you can't respond to properly, being asked to cut corners to fit in more clients, and the constant feeling of an unmanageable level of work.

Here are some examples of the adaptive responses that we see in burnout and why the body and brain develop them:

What You Might Notice Happening Inside You (Adaptive Response)	Why This Happens
Thoughts or images that keep interrupting your day (known as intrusive thoughts) about things that have happened (e.g., replaying conversations or texts you've sent)	Brain trying to make sense of it all to ensure it doesn't happen again
Being on guard and wary of bad things happening	Brain preempting what could go wrong next
Body feeling on edge and unable to relax	Body watching for cues of danger and being ready to act on this quickly
Emotions shutting off (emotional detachment or zoning out)	Body switching off from intense emotions because it can't act on them effectively anyway and they feel too painful
Sidestepping things that remind you of the excessive demands (such as avoiding opening your emails, not responding to messages, or avoiding socializing)	Brain reducing the feeling of being under attack again and keeping the feeling of helplessness at bay

THE TRAUMA OF BURNOUT

What You Might Notice Happening Inside You (Adaptive Response)	Why This Happens
Urges to people-please (doing what others want, putting others' needs first, or never saying "no" to demands)	Brain trying to avoid further criticism, rejection, or making others angry
Urges to prove yourself (excessive striving to achieve or perfectionist behaviors)	Brain trying to avoid feeling inferior or rejected

So far, we have looked at where the physical and psychological issues in burnout can arise from:

1. excessive allostatic load from chronic stress, *and*
2. difficulty resting and replenishing in a restorative way, *and*
3. an understandable adaptive nervous-system response to the demands and little-t traumas of life.

However, there are four more ways in which the external pressures contributing to burnout overlap with trauma:

1. Unmet needs
2. Violated boundaries
3. Insufficient social support
4. Feeling of being trapped

Let's take a look at each of these in turn.

Unmet Needs

Trauma is what happens to a person where there is too much too soon, too much for too long, *or not enough for too long.*

—Peg Duros and Dee Crowley,
"The Body Comes to Therapy Too"

We have already explored "too much" and "too long" (inescapable stress), so this definition is an invitation to explore "not enough for too long," referring to the unmet needs of the human nervous system. When our core human needs go unmet, our nervous systems respond as though under threat. This is called "trauma of omission." It is harder to spot this type of trauma because there isn't a moment something happened but rather a chronic absence or denial of experiences that are essential for human well-being.

In their book *A Straight Talking Introduction to the Power Threat Meaning Framework*, psychologists and leading thinkers on human distress Mary Boyle and Lucy Johnstone summarize the core human needs as follows:

- To be safe, valued, and cared for in our earliest relationships
- To have a sense of security and belonging in a family, friendship, or social group
- To feel safe and secure in our physical environments
- To form intimate relationships and partnerships
- To experience and manage a range of emotions
- To feel valued and effective in our family or social roles
- To have some control over important parts of our lives, including our bodies and emotions
- To meet basic physical and material needs for ourselves and our dependents
- To experience some sense of justice or fairness about our circumstances
- To make connections to the natural world
- To engage in meaningful activities and, more generally, to have a sense of hope, meaning, and purpose in our lives

A well-known model for this is Maslow's hierarchy which places the basic needs for survival, such as physiological requirements (food, water, and safety) at the base, with belonging and self-esteem needs following once those are met.

When our needs are met at all levels, we feel fulfilled and content, but the theory posits that we cannot focus on the needs of the higher levels unless the ones below are being adequately met. However, humans have developed ways to "cheat" the levels, jumping over the hurdle of unmet needs to try to find fulfillment at the higher levels of the pyramid through using tools that temporarily bring relief and mask distress, such as emotional eating, busying onself to distract, using drugs, overachieving, and so on. Of course, the difficulty with this is that these are often misaligned with what you really want for yourself. They can also exacerbate burnout.

Many people can miss just how poorly or tenuously their basic needs are being met in the present or were met in the past. It's also very common to misunderstand the extent of the negative impact this has on humans.

Violated Boundaries

Burnout is overwhelming and boundaries are the cure.

—Nedra Glover Tawwab, therapist and social worker

A second feature in trauma is a violation of someone's boundaries. A boundary is an imaginary wall that separates you from others to allow you to feel safe and in control. Within that boundary wall, you can keep the things that are important to you, such as your values, time, body, and opinions.

When someone crosses your boundary wall without your permission, this sets off your amber mode, particularly anger or annoyance—an emotional response designed to tell you that this wasn't OK! If it happens repeatedly, or you feel powerless to assert where your boundary is, then this can be experienced as traumatic, especially if physically removing yourself from the situation isn't possible either.

Example of traumatic boundary violations include physical or sexual assault (physical-boundary violations) and emotional abuse—a violation of emotional boundaries, such as emotional blackmail (when you are made to feel bad for your opinion or values), bullying, or chipping away at someone's self-worth.

In the situation of burnout, there is typically at least one of these boundary breaches:

- **Personal-Time Violations:** Being expected to check emails outside working hours, working longer hours than you should, or not feeling able to take lunch or coffee breaks.
- **Emotional-Boundary Violations:** Being made to feel guilty for sticking to your paid work hours, turning down extra shifts, or feeling lazy if you take a break. Policies like compassionate leave often allow between three and five paid days following an upsetting life event with managers' discretion required for further time off. The reality is, however, that in many big life events three to five days would only allow you to process the initial shock, so it is emotionally invalidating to be expected to be ready to work at the end of that time.
- **Moral-Boundary Violations:** Being asked to do things that don't align with your values and feeling like you have no choice. An example of this is a teacher being expected to take on too many pupils or do too much paperwork to teach effectively, or a nurse feeling unable to respond to a distressed patient's requests because there are more pressing emergencies. This has been a big issue in the NHS, particularly during COVID-19, when many difficult decisions were being made quickly that went against the staff's training and moral values.

Insufficient Social Support

Trauma is not what happens to us. It's what we hold inside in the absence of an empathic witness.

—Peter Levine, therapist and author

The third way in which burnout and trauma overlap is where there is an absence of support or understanding from others about the situation. Research shows that big-T traumatic incidents like national disasters tend to have lower incidents of PTSD than those where there are no witnesses or where there is a prevailing victim-blaming mentality, such as "they brought it on themselves." This causes a sense of shame, prevents verbal processing of the event, and leads to withdrawal from potential support.

How does this idea translate to burnout? Busyness, stress, and anxiety have become so accepted and normal that many people worry that they are burdening others if they complain or believe they are weak if they ask for a much-needed break. We are shamed for our basic human needs for rest in micro ways. Some examples include: raised eyebrows when we log off at the actual time our shift ends rather than staying online, and quips that make us feel like this is just the way it is, like, "Welcome to parent-hood" or "Sleeping's cheating."

These can chip away at us, making it hard to stick to our bound-aries and reducing the likelihood that we will seek help. They stop us from listening to the signs of stress and recognizing that we are entitled to more. For example, I saw recently a cry-for-help post on a local parenting Facebook group; the parent obviously being overwhelmed and stressed. The comments in reply were all varia-tions of "I feel you" or "Being a mom to toddlers is tough"; no one was able to offer solutions of change or suggestions for where to get support, suggesting that learned helplessness can go beyond the individual and become a group mentality.

We could go one step further and consider this as a form of gaslighting. We *know* it's not possible to work full time in addi-tion to being the perfect attentive parent, going to the gym three times a week, and eating freshly prepared meals every night. But the messages we get from the world around us (compounded by marketing and social media) make it all seem possible. We then doubt our feelings that it's unrealistic and believe there's something wrong with us because we are struggling to cope.

LEARNED HELPLESSNESS

In the 1960s, a famous experiment was carried out by psychologist and educator Martin Seligman and colleagues. In part one of the study, individual dogs were harnessed to a shuttle box where they were exposed to electric shocks. In Group A, the dogs could escape the shocks by pressing a lever; however, with Group B the shocks would stop and start at random, meaning those dogs had no control over their adverse situation.

In part two of the study, the same dogs were introduced to a new shuttle box, where they could jump over a low partition into a second section to escape the shocks. The Group A dogs quickly learned to jump to safety, but the ones in Group B didn't. They lay down and whined, giving in without realizing they now had some control over their situation. This giving-up behavior became known as "learned helplessness."

It was possible to modify the response of the Group B dogs with an intervention: If the researchers physically lifted them and started to move their legs, then they could learn how to get to safety on their own. However, this intervention had to be repeated at least twice for them to realize that they now had some control over their situation. Alternative techniques, such as visual demonstrations, threats, and rewards, failed to overcome the learned helplessness; the dogs required the physical movement to get going.

The take-home from this for burnout is that it's not your fault if you feel helpless, because the chances are high that you have had limited opportunities to control your adverse situation. However, physical movement and focusing on aspects of your situation that *are* within your control *can* break the pattern. But you cannot do something once and hope that that will be the fix. You need to repeat the healthy patterns continually. Humans are more likely to stick with behaviors required to feel better when they understand themselves and the neuroscience, which is why the first chunk of this book focuses on why this behavior occurs while the later sections explain how to address and fix it.

Feeling of Being Trapped

The origin of trauma is the inability to move (i.e., the immobilization response).... Trauma is characterized by being stuck.

—Bessel van der Kolk, Dutch psychiatrist and author

Imagine you are practicing tennis and using a tennis-ball machine to fire shots for you. When the shots come at a good pace, you can return them and be ready for the next one. But if the speed is too fast, you become frenzied and have to rush to reach each ball. Now imagine a second machine is placed next to the first... This is what real life is often like with multiple demands from family and work. With so many balls coming at you and nowhere to escape, the urge, eventually, is to curl into a ball yourself to minimize the impact of the hits.

When external pressures are too much to escape from or have eroded our boundaries and squeezed out any social support, then where can we turn to for help? In an inescapable situation, where our nervous systems' first line of defense—fight or flight—has gone on for too long without success, our body does the next best things to stay safe: "freeze," "appease," or, as a last-ditch attempt, shut down completely which is known as "flop." These three reactions are a sign that the nervous system is tipping into its trauma response. It can also lead to the phenomenon known as learned helplessness: a "what's-the-point-of-trying?" mentality and giving-up behaviors (see the box on page 55).

A prey animal in the state of flop can be seen to stop breathing for up to a minute, making it appear lifeless. This may seem like a strange reaction in the face of danger, but at the point of apparent defeat when faced with a predator it is the best way to avoid injury or death. Without the thrill of the chase igniting the predator's sympathetic nervous system, it loses interest and may also take its eye off the ball, allowing the prey to reanimate and run off to safety.

In humans, flopping can involve dissociation—a mild version of which is daydreaming or zoning out—when it can look like you're not listening or paying attention. This is often accompanied by a physical heaviness, like everything is an effort as well as being emotionally detached from (or less bothered about) friends, family, and hobbies, like you're just going through the motions on autopilot. These are all familiar signs of burnout.

This is the red mode. What is happening in your nervous system at this point? How is it different than amber, and why does this make you feel so stuck? To answer these questions, we need to visit the oldest part of the nervous system. Let's move to the next chapter.

Chapter 3

RED MODE: WHY WE SHUT DOWN IN BURNOUT

Having built his business from scratch, Scott felt unable to put any of the moving parts down for even a moment. He struggled to trust that anyone would do the different tasks to the high standard he expected and, consequently, he wore all the hats (marketer, accountant, technician, and CEO) all at once, meaning he never reached the end of a to-do list. While he had managed to close a deal recently, it had been in the pipeline for almost a year. Even though it looked like a marker of success to anyone looking in, he knew his creativity and output had nose-dived. This was discomforting, and, moreover, had set off his inner critic with a vengeance: "You're useless, you're an imposter, you don't deserve a break..." He had thought that being his own boss would give him freedom, but it turned out he wasn't the compassionate boss he needed for this level of uncertainty and stress. With no one to turn to for practical or moral support, Scott felt trapped.

So far, we have been moving in and out of green and amber modes—the relaxed green mode when the ventral vagal part of the parasympathetic nervous system takes charge, and the energized amber mode when the sympathetic nervous system takes charge. The third and last mode is red when the dorsal vagal nerve takes charge. To get a sense of how this branch of your nervous system functions, think of a turtle retreating into its shell when it feels threatened, immobilized, and hiding away until the threat has passed. Even though our nervous systems developed newer options for responding to threats, we still have this original, more primitive response in our repertoires.

Scott, as previously mentioned, felt trapped. For over a year, he had been doing the work of four people to build up his business. He was worn out with no end in sight. There was no one above him to tell him he should take a vacation or to turn to for help, and he didn't feel able to share the extent of his stress and anxiety with friends or family for fear of being seen as weak. The neuroscience shows that when we are faced with continual external stresses or pressures with no option of escaping, our nervous systems take the next best available step, namely dorsal vagal shutdown: red mode.

RED MODE WHEN WE *AREN'T* UNDER THREAT

It's important to know that each of the three branches of your nervous system can operate on its own but also in tandem with each other; that is to say, two modes can be online at once in what is known as blended states.

There is a deeply restorative level of rest that occurs when green and red modes are engaged simultaneously. A day spent resting or a night of deep sleep gives you a good dose of this type of replenishment, meaning that your cells have had a chance to repair from their wear and tear, your digestive system can settle back into a healthy pattern, and your muscles can release their pent-up tension.

We can, of course, rest in a more social manner, which happens when the green mode is in the driving seat, such as hanging out with friends. This may help us feel connected and soothed but doesn't provide the same level of physical restoration. Deep rest that comes from the blend of red and green modes is more of an inward, solitary activity. We are choosing to temporarily disconnect from life's pressures and social world in a way that feels good and safe; we become still and the nonessential workings of the body can be given a thorough break.

Here are some examples of times when my clients have described being more able to get into a deeply restorative rest state. See if any of these resonates with you:

- During or after a warm bath
- In nature
- On vacation (usually at least a few days in)
- After strenuous exercise
- With pets
- Reading a book
- Meditating or spiritual practices
- Daydreaming or pleasantly zoning out (looks like "doing nothing")

This type of rest is not only essential for our day-to-day well-being, but, after a highly stressful event, a restorative rest can mitigate against mental-health difficulties becoming more pronounced (such as meeting diagnostic criteria for PTSD).

If we relate this to burnout, we can see how modern-day living sets us up to be almost permanently "on," preventing this deep level of rest despite the strong need to recover from the constant barrage of stress and demands. We may *think* that we are resting when we are watching TV, but, if we are also booking a trip on our phone or refreshing our social media newsfeed for #insert-trend-name-here at the same time, we are actually in green and amber modes—feeling safe and engaged but also mobilized and taking action.

We are also conditioned to feel guilty for those moments when we are "doing nothing." If we were to rebrand "doing nothing" as "doing deeply restorative rest," then that might help us to lean into those moments.

How Deep Rest Is Important to Our Sense of Identity
And something else magical happens when we allow ourselves to "do nothing." Brain scans show that a surprising amount of activity occurs in our brains during this time when our minds are wandering freely. This is called the default mode network (DMN). The DMN is thought to be important in the processing of emotions and linking back to autobiographical memories, all essential to our sense of identity—something that can feel lost in burnout.

RED MODE WHEN WE *ARE* UNDER THREAT
The threat version of the dorsal vagal system lights up when our attempts to escape from the threat with the energized amber mode are blocked or have been fruitless. The dorsal reaction is one of disconnection and immobilization. When we move into this red mode, the body has sensed that the threat is too big to fight or escape from and that the most likely way of surviving is by "playing dead." This is also known

as flop and, as mentioned earlier, in burnout it may not look like a physical flopping down but more of a mental zoning out or disengagement that is more subtle, albeit just as problematic given that it stops us from being properly present in many activities.

Imagine having a tricky conversation with a friend or family member that goes badly. This may start off with attempts to talk reasonably and to see each other's viewpoint, but, if you have opposing views and cannot agree, the conversation may stop feeling collaborative and become heated. This is a sign that both of your systems are shifting into their amber sympathetic nervous systems of fight or flight. This is an energized place where your body feels fired up and you get urges to quickly fix the problem. This can cause the talking to get louder and an increase in gesticulating. If there still isn't a satisfactory resolution, then eventually your body might shift into its final gear: red mode, or dorsal shutdown. Now you just want to give up. The conversation seems pointless, and you find yourself saying things like "Do whatever you want, then," as you feel resigned and lose your motivation.

This is an example of how our nervous systems can shift gear from amber to red mode in the course of a conversation. Burnout recovery is not about avoiding red or amber modes completely. The aim, rather, is to support the nervous system to move fluidly through the gears again throughout the day. I'll provide the tools in Chapter 5 to regulate from amber and red back to green for you to do with confidence.

WHAT DOES RED MODE IN BURNOUT LOOK LIKE?

Here are some common signs that you have dipped into your red mode and why.

What Is Happening?	How You Might Recognize This	Why It Happens
Zoning out or feeling detached from what's happening around you	Others say they've already told you information, but you haven't been able to remember it; or they think you seem distracted and like you're not listening.	This is a mild form of dissociation. Dissociation is a way for the brain and body to cope with intensity by disconnecting from the information available to the five senses.
Feeling flat or experiencing a general numbing of all emotions	You appear almost indifferent or unable to enjoy things that are happening in the moment. This can be experienced as empathy-distress fatigue. Your face may look flat and unanimated.	Emotions like anxiety and anger (in amber mode) bring an energy that allows you to act in ways to stay safe. If you've moved out of amber, then these emotional strategies have been blocked so have been fruitless, and to feel these without being able to take steps can be distressing. As such, your systems can try to keep you safe from feeling with an emotional numbing.
Feeling drained of energy	Your body may feel heavy and tired. You have no motivation.	Red mode is all about conservation of energy and immobilization.
Withdrawal from help or others	Wanting to give up and thoughts that sound like, "What's the point?" or "This is useless"; turning down social events or avoiding approaching people when opportunities arise naturally (e.g., at school or at the water cooler).	Asking for support from others can be seen as a vulnerability or a fear of burdening people so will often be avoided at all costs, especially because to have reached red mode means you already feel at your most threatened and vulnerable. Moreover, the idea that support from others could help may be hard to imagine.
Autopilot function switches on	Just going through the motions or agreeing with others without a full connection as to what's happening.	With the frontal cortex and higher-brain functioning offline, you are only left with access to the more basic brain functioning that allows you to carry out behaviors that have been rehearsed to the point of being ingrained habits (more on the autopilot ability on page 65).

What Is Happening?	How You Might Recognize This	Why It Happens
You have an impaired ability to think clearly or imaginatively and you're unable to solve problems.	Problems feel huge and insurmountable. You may not be able to picture how things could be different or break things down into steps to overcome it. You may also make more mistakes, like turning up to the meeting at the wrong time, burning the dinner, or booking the wrong train.	This is the point at which your functional IQ is at its lowest because the rational, thinking part of your brain is not online.
Your emotional mind is making all the decisions.	You get irritable or overwhelmed by decisions that may have felt easy in the past, such as what to make for dinner. Or you are impulsive and make decisions you wouldn't typically make when feeling calm.	Rational decision-making requires access to the rational thinking part of the brain which is not online at this time. Impulsive decision-making is due to an avoidance and wanting to escape.
Your language and communication centers are functioning poorly.	Difficulty communicating effectively (e.g., finding words or being eloquent) or taking on board what others are saying. For example, one person in clinical burnout woke up one morning unable to speak.	The language center (Broca's area) is housed in the frontal lobes which, as already explained, is not the part of the brain in the driving seat when in red mode.
You're unable to switch tasks easily.	You may procrastinate or struggle to initiate the next task in your day: for example, finding yourself glued to the computer or standing in the shower until it runs cold and you are jolted back.	Moments of transition require energy and cognitive power to make decisions, all of which run low in red mode.

Autopilot During Burnout

How is it that we can manage to carry out seemingly complex tasks like cooking, driving, or even teaching classes when we are in red mode—feeling disconnected and shut down?

"Just going through the motions" is something that many people in burnout are familiar with. Being on autopilot like this means that you are managing to do the tasks that are expected of you without really thinking about them deeply or feeling connected to them. You may struggle to remember completing a task or feel overwhelmed if a seemingly small obstacle gets in the way of carrying it out—for example, a roadblock on your usual drive home may throw you into a spin.

Essentially, this type of functioning relies on procedural memory that is instrumental in helping us to form habits. I can make myself a cup of tea without having to think through each step: get out a cup, pour water into the kettle, turn it on, get a teabag…Procedural memory is housed deep inside the brain (the basal ganglia), so that the brain can free up thinking space. This allows me to listen to the radio or have a conversation while making the tea. Conversely, new skills require our prefrontal cortex, an energy-intensive part of the brain, to be online. This is why new-skill acquisition is tricky when we are feeling burned-out, because the frontal lobes aren't functioning optimally and we have little energy to draw on. We need to shift gear from red mode (thaw out from immobilization and energy conservation) to get our frontal cortex fired up again.

In burnout, you may have become skilled at relying on this deep, procedural memory to go through the motions, and this is why your burnout is so well masked from both yourself and others. Signs that this is the case include struggling to incorporate new ideas (say, during a training day at work) or remembering the steps in new procedures.

Panic, Stress, Anxiety, and Freeze

"Panic," "stress," and "anxiety" are terms people often use to describe the human freeze response. It's frequently assumed that freeze is the full dorsal vagal shutdown of red mode described previously, but actually the freeze state is generally considered a blended state of both red *and* amber modes together. This means you have the pent-up energy from the sympathetic system urging you to move, but you feel stuck and unable to break out of this.

"Functional freeze" refers to this stuckness in relation to over-working, where you work through your needs to rest, eat, and get comfortable. You appear functional and might be fooling those around you, but you are really on autopilot and disconnected from them.

People-Pleasing

This also needs its own section because it is the term commonly used for another survival response known as "appease" or "fawn." Also a blended state of red and amber, fawn is when we mimic the social-engagement system of green mode to try to feel safe: smiling and nodding, agreeing with others, or trying to preempt their needs so they don't get upset, while all the time feeling numb or apprehensive, hypervigilant for their responses ("Was that a smile or a smirk?" or "They're not really listening to me"). You may feel like you are treading on eggshells or racing through thoughts of what you should do or say next. Some people operate at this level so successfully that even the people closest to them might be misled. Unfortunately, the positive social cues you're giving off in the fawn response can mask how much you're struggling.

People-pleasing is a common response to early life relationship stresses in our family or friendships. Of course, it can also be a big reason for your burnout where the emphasis on keeping others happy has left no time to tend to your own needs.

Moreover, the depletion of your resources through burnout may exacerbate this people-pleasing pattern because it is your default autonomic response to threat. We will explore people-pleasing in more detail in Chapter 8.

HOW TO IDENTIFY THE STATE OF YOUR NERVOUS SYSTEM

Bringing all three branches of the nervous system together, the summary table indicates how you may feel, act, think, and behave depending on which mode you are in.

	Green Ventral Vagal (at Rest)	Amber Sympathetic (Mobilized)	Red Dorsal Vagal (Immobilized)
What This Mode Is About	Socially engaged and present; rest and recuperation	Survival motivations: energy to get to safety Non-survival motivations: energy to get resources like food, a mate, or social status	Survival motivation: to immobilize when danger persists and amber has failed to create safety Non-survival motivation: deep rest
Possible Emotions and How This Feels	Content Calm Access to emotions that connect us to other humans, like compassion, sadness, or empathy	Fight: Agitated Angry Cynical Irritable Flight: Anxious Panicky Overwhelmed Worried	Empty Ashamed Numb Helpless Despair Hopeless Indifferent
Bodily Sensations	May notice "business-as-usual" sensations like digestion, hunger cues, or feeling hot or cold Light and free	Heart racing Breathing faster Blood pressure goes up Restless feeling Muscles tense up Digestion slows down (needing the bathroom, getting butterflies, or feeling nauseous)	Fatigue May feel pains in back, shoulders, and head Body feels heavy or sluggish

	Green Ventral Vagal (at Rest)	Amber Sympathetic (Mobilized)	Red Dorsal Vagal (Immobilized)
Mental (Cognitive) Abilities	Able to focus on problems without becoming overwhelmed Can access creative and imaginative thought Feeling generally capable Can accurately read facial expressions and body language of others Thought that follows a logic or access to abstract ideas is possible	Racing Haphazard Narrow focus on problems and fears for the future	Foggy brain Struggling to think of solutions Making mistakes Lack of thoughts on how to initiate action Lack of imaginative or inspirational thoughts Feeling like people are too much for you Wanting to be left in peace Avoidance of decision-making (feels too much) Communication difficulties
Thinking Styles	*I'll be OK* (keeping things in perspective) *I need to do X to feel better* (ability to plan and self-care) *I'm doing a good enough job* (connection to internal resources)	*This is urgent* (emotional reasoning) *I'm going to fail* (overestimating the likelihood something bad will happen) *What if…* *This is completely awful* (catastrophizing) *Nothing helps* (black-and-white thinking)	*I'm useless* (self-attacking) *It's all hopeless* (pessimism) *They think I'm useless* (mind-reading)
Behaviors	Unhurried Seeking out connection or feeling peaceful with being in your own company	Chaotic Urgent Rushing Impatient Restless Reassurance seeking Trying to fix the problem ASAP	Withdrawing socially (this may be declining invitations or if you are in social situations being less socially engaged with the people around you—for example, closed body language or reduced eye contact) Moving slowly Doing actions by rote because you're on autopilot

An important skill for climbing out of burnout is being able to recognize the different aspects of your nervous system—that is, how your different gears feel when you are in each one. It can be hard to recognize without practice; in moments when you get caught up in the content of your negative thoughts and emotions, this becomes all-consuming and it's difficult to think about the processes of your nervous system at play. The easiest way to start is to bring to mind a recent time when you felt one of the modes come online. This should allow you to note down the components of your experience (your thoughts, feelings, emotions, and behaviors), while still feeling one step removed so you don't get pulled into the full force of the emotions again as you do so.

Use the questions in the following table to start exploring your own responses. Mapping all three will help you to recognize where you are in your nervous system, as this is not always obvious. The body responses in amber mode are loud—it can feel like the body is shouting at you (heart thumping or feeling hot)—but in green mode this is more of a whisper, so locating where you feel contentedness in your body will allow you to be more receptive to it.

	Green	Amber	Red
What is happening?	Example: walking home from work	Example: receiving an email from a client telling me their order hasn't arrived	Example: seeing a photo of my friends all socializing on Instagram without me
	Your turn:	Your turn:	Your turn:

	Green	Amber	Red
Where are you? Describe your surroundings in detail.	Example: the park; sunny autumn day; people reading on benches and kids on their bikes	Example: cooking dinner and checking my work phone between chopping veggies; radio on; kids watching TV in the living room, so a lot of background noise	Example: alone, watching TV, and scrolling through social media
	Your turn:	Your turn:	Your turn:
Who are you with (if anyone)?	Example: no one except others around you	Example: no one in the kitchen; the kids nearby	Example: no one
	Your turn:	Your turn:	Your turn:
What else was going on just before this? For amber and red, this helps you to understand your triggers.	Example: I had finished work—nothing too stressful had happened today though; I hadn't finished my to-do list but had left a clear action to start on tomorrow, so felt "tidy"	Example: I arrived home from picking up my daughter from her football practice; I needed to start dinner quickly, as the kids were getting grumpy and hungry	Example: I had been scrolling through social media for half an hour, half-watching a TV show but having to rewind every so often as I kept missing important moments
	Your turn:	Your turn:	Your turn:
What did you feel in your body?	Calm, slowing down; warmth in stomach	Example: agitated and hot; heart raced as I saw the email	Example: shock followed by heaviness and slumping over in the chair
	Your turn:	Your turn:	Your turn:

	Green	Amber	Red
What thoughts accompanied this?	Example: my thoughts meandered gently as I walked about—various topics, like what to cook for dinner and what to watch on TV	Example: I need to get this sorted quickly before the complaint escalates	Example: they don't like me; no one likes me; I'm so lonely; what's the point of trying when I'm treated like this?
	Your turn:	Your turn:	Your turn:
What behaviors did you do? Or, to put it another way, what urges did you get?	Example: I was content to walk at an unhurried pace; I had an urge to knock on my friend's door as I walked by, but she wasn't home which was OK	Example: an urge to reply immediately rather than go through the client case logically to compose a more measured response tomorrow	Example: I sat and scrolled compulsively for another hour or so; I stopped paying any proper attention to either the phone or the TV
	Your turn:	Your turn:	Your turn:

Keep in mind that while your gears might feel stuck in survival mode and you might at times feel as though your car has completely stalled, you are still the one behind the steering wheel. Becoming aware of your body's thoughts, feelings, and behaviors in the previously described way is the first step in starting to take back control.

Chapter 4

HOW TO FEEL SAFE

———————

Anika's work environment (a county hospital ward) was hectic. From the moment she stepped on to the unit there were tasks that felt urgent and multiple people making demands of her. This was a big part of why she had slipped from stressed to burned out—the highly demanding context and the fact that she felt she had no choice but to go through the entire shift without pause. Stepping back from the busyness for a break felt impossible because the work was so pressing all the time. When I asked her when there were moments of social connection with others she could only really think of the connections with patients, all of which were emotionally intense due to the nature of their illnesses. Her frenetic behavior had finally culminated in early morning panic attacks before work when she would become frozen and unable to do anything. As she came around from these, she would feel disconnected from everything, driving in to work on autopilot with a sense of dread of the day to come.

If your gearbox is stuck in the survival red and amber modes, you need to learn how to get it working fluidly again and, importantly, how to get more access to green.

We cannot come back to our resting green mode if we don't feel safe enough. Our nervous systems need to assess the current level of risk and perceive that we are safe before returning us to our less guarded green mode.

Anxiety tools and ventral vagal exercises can be helpful and have found popularity on social media following a trend in sharing ventral vagal hacks. However, it is only possible to inhibit our amber and red modes and enjoy a restorative spell in green mode when we also feel safe. It takes context as well as tools (which I give you in Chapter 5). And as we saw in Chapter 2, our environments are rarely conducive to feeling safe, because our green mode is being hindered by the constant demands of our busy and highly stimulating modern world. So how do we override this?

We can start to improve our sense of safety by making small adjustments that are in sympathy with our neuroception, the body's inbuilt surveillance system that at a preconscious level is always watching for signs of safety and threats. For immediate minor adjustments we can experiment with glimmers.

GLIMMERS—THE OPPOSITE OF TRIGGERS

While triggers are stimuli that push us into threat modes, glimmers are moments that have the potential to regulate back into green, but they only work if we notice them. Noticing glimmers is not easy when we are rushing and overwhelmed, so we need to lean into them to secure their goodness. The boxes in this chapter capture glimmer ideas that have been shown in research and clinical practice to be helpful for many.

The concept of glimmers comes from Deb Dana, a licensed consultant therapist who has skillfully translated polyvagal theory into therapy-friendly ideas. Dana also outlines the three Cs of safety: elements of our environment that provide the cues our nervous system need to figure out how safe we are. They are:

- C for context
- C for connection
- C for choice

C for Context
This is the information about our current situation that helps us understand what is happening and whether it is safe or not. It includes the who, what, how, and why of what is going on, although we also draw on our preexisting ideas about ourselves and the world to help make sense of this.

A smell of smoke will set off our internal alarms, unless we have been told that a bonfire has been lit in the neighbor's garden, in which case this contextualizing information reassures us that we are safe. When something about the situation doesn't "add up," we become suspicious (i.e., our threat response gets alerted that this could be a sign of trouble).

Our nervous system will default to amber mode if it doesn't have enough of a sense of safety from a situation to allow it to stand down. So many of our behaviors are about understanding our contexts, especially as we try to make choices that impact our days. Context-seeking behaviors might include checking the weather to decide what we should wear; looking up symptoms on the internet to learn more about them; or investigating where a new, unfamiliar smell is coming from. When we lack the cues of safety, our amber mode responds with an urgency to find them, causing strong urges to do more of these behaviors. This is where they can tip into reassurance seeking from other people ("Did I sound OK?") or triple-checking things (such as news or travel updates or looking up where you're going on Google Maps). This can set off a vicious cycle of increasing focus on the uncertainty, thus increasing anxiety and increasing urges to check.

The reason we prefer routines and familiar places is that they reduce the need for context-seeking behaviors and help us to feel confident and safe. Routine also allows us to know when it will be safe to shut down for the day and rest without negative repercussions. When we are faced with uncertainty or novelty, our nervous systems must risk-assess them. This results in anxiety, as our nervous systems move into standby in case action is required. Even pleasant life events create uncertainty—moving, going on vacation, and starting a new job still bring a sense of the unknown.

But certainty is not the only important thing here. A safe context is also one that provides us with the physical space, permission, and opportunities to slow down and rest. Sadly, modern life doesn't make this accessible. Instead of environments that encourage downtime, we are expected to be reactive and available 24–7, which is reflected in our physical space, too. As an example, when I worked in the NHS there was nowhere to sit and eat my lunch inside the building that wasn't in a work zone or in front of a desk. The kitchen only had space for two people standing up. That was it. So my options in a rainy break time were to sit in front of all the work I hadn't finished or in front of others hard at work—neither of which was conducive to rest!

SPATIAL CONTEXT

People may have an innate visual preference for moderately complex, savannah-like environments because these areas signal both safety and nourishment.
—Alexander Coburn, 2017, "Buildings, Beauty, and the Brain"

Our sensory systems prefer stimuli from the natural world. In his work on the human nervous system and building design, researcher

Alex Coburn found that man-made spaces that imitate certain elements of nature support good well-being. Movements that mimic nature (such as leaves gently blowing in the wind or water flowing), the use of natural materials like wood and plants, and plenty of natural light all have a positive effect on us. Humans instinctively prefer spaces that replicate the features of an environment that would have enabled our ancestors to survive and thrive.

Coburn's research shows that three key aspects of our environment make us feel safe and secure:

- **Fluency:** an orderliness that helps us to navigate the space safely
- **Fascination:** interesting scenery which gives us options for hiding from predators and finding food
- **Hygge or Hominess:** opportunities to get cozy, enabling us to nurture our connections with others and also safely rest

If the spaces you spend most time in give you these three things, you are providing your nervous system with a head start in feeling safe. An example of this is the cozy feeling you get in a nook in a coffee shop, surrounded by cushions, or why many people feel better when their homes are tidy and orderly.

HOW OUR SYSTEMS ABSORB INFORMATION FROM OUR CONTEXT

Our environmental context affects us through our senses and bodies. If the ventral vagal nerve is stimulated in a soothing way, this will have a calming effect. This nerve has endings most densely clustered in the top half of the body:

- **Ears:** Sound is an important way for our nervous systems to search for cues of safety with lower-frequency sounds reminding us of predators. When we feel unsafe, we become hypersensitive to background noise. Our ear muscles tighten and we are less able to tune in to any human voice above it.

- **Eyes:** When we are alert, our pupils dilate to scan for dangers. They seek out cues of safety often found in familiar faces, colors of nature, and patterns that look regular and predictable. Our eyes also naturally scan from left to right when we walk or move through the world to take in our environments. Research now shows this left–right, bilateral movement allows us to stay alert but dampens down the threat center of the brain enough to stop us from becoming frozen or avoidant.

- **Skin:** Stimulation around the areas of the body where the ventral vagal nerves are clustered can be soothing—warmth and cold as well as tactile touch. However, human touch is particularly important because this releases oxytocin. Skin-to-skin contact is one of the most powerful ways of releasing oxytocin; this includes self-touch, such as holding areas of your body that are linked to your ventral vagal nerve (see page 93).

- **Movement of Our Bodies:** Each autonomic state, be it in green, amber, or red mode, is associated with a level of energy and movement. Increasing energy levels can therefore be used as regulation. Responding to your moment-to-moment needs is therapeutic and interpreted by your system as safe, particularly when you move parts of the body associated with the ventral vagal nerve. For example, slowly turning your head from side to side activates the ventral vagal nerve of green mode.

BLOCKS TO FINDING SAFE CONTEXTS IN MODERN LIFE

Part of the difficulty in modern life is that the necessary areas of our bodies are not being stimulated in calming ways. Life is noisy and busy which causes our heart rate to increase and our muscles to tense for action. Here are some examples of how modern contexts keep our bodies in a state of readiness.

- **Auditory:** In modern life, there is a lot of background sound and electronic noises that our ancestors were not exposed to (vehicles reversing, the fridge beeping, city noises of traffic, and alarms). These can make it hard to tune in to the meaningful sounds of safety, like human voices. Earplugs that dampen down noise have become a popular way of coping with this type of overstimulation and might be worth exploring if you feel particularly susceptible to this.
- **Visual:** Witnessing violent or environmentally catastrophic events on social media and the TV, whether fictional or real, has become normal to us, but these are strong cues of danger for our nervous systems. The same applies if we have only limited access to calming scenery because we live in built-up environments or to friendly faces if we work in isolation.
- **Movement:** Moving appropriately for our nervous systems can be difficult if it doesn't fit with a work or school routine, a lot of which can mean being sedentary for long periods. Extended time spent staring straight ahead at screens means that the ventral vagal nerve in the neck and head and the bilateral movements of the eyes aren't being exercised regularly. Simple stretches and looking around help with this.
- **Space:** Many modern urban developments adhere to the concept of "form follows function," which means that the functionality— or fluency—of the space is prioritized but hygge and fascination are not considered. Buildings that give a sense of space, use natural materials, provide variety, create community spaces for connection, and spark our creativity are, sadly, a dwindling feature of both our residential and workplace environments.
- **Lack of Dedicated Relaxing Spaces:** Home was traditionally considered our safe space, but in reality it tends to be full of reminders about all the jobs we've not yet done, and, for anyone who lives in a busy family environment, it might not be a

peaceful space. Now that more people work from home, boundaries between home and work are blurred. When I explored this concept of a safe, relaxing environment with Anika, even her bedroom didn't feel like the refuge she needed because her work laptop lived by her bed: Something many people do either because space is limited or simply because of habit. And this is true of phones as well. The constant access to the world that we have via our screens means there is always some noisy stimulation disrupting our bodies' ability to tune in to cues of safety.

FINDING SAFE CONTEXTS IN MODERN LIFE

Think of the locations where you *are* able to feel safe and calm. If you find this tricky, consider places you are drawn to and what it is about them that makes you feel good. How else can you bring more of this into your day? Even in micro ways. If, for example, you have a favorite relaxing view from a window, can you drink your morning coffee there?

Many people, when they feel overwhelmed, intuitively sense that getting out into the natural world will help. But there is also research to support it: Blue spaces like coastlines and rivers improve our feelings of creativity and calm; forest bathing—the term given to mindfully spending time soaking up the calming effect of woodlands—improves the effects of stress linked to technology anxiety.

Of course, it's not always possible to take ourselves out into nature, and with over half the world's population living in an urban environment, we need alternatives. Fortunately, we can get the same effect through other means. For example, a study into still images carried out by Japanese researchers in 2017 showed that spending just ninety seconds looking at an image of forests has a calming effect on subjects' physiologies.

This also works with images on screen. *Guardian* video game editor Keza MacDonald publicly shared how her escape into video game *The Legend of Zelda: Breath of the Wild* helped her navigate the emotional intensity of life with a newborn. This game is renowned for its breathtaking scenery and, although gaming traditionally has a bad reputation for mental health because of a focus on violent games, many offer positive stimulation, too. My household has a particular liking for slow-paced TV shows involving famous comedians talking casually in natural settings as they fish, take a ramble through nature, or paint.

GLIMMERS: FINDING MOMENTS OF SAFETY AT HOME AND WORK

Where to Look for Glimmers	Home	Work
Sights		
Sounds		
Smells		
Textures		
Tastes		

Which of these create calm for you?

- **Sights:** posters, video game scenery, photos, views, the garden, your pet, meaningful items that help you feel good, decluttering to create more space and orderliness, or a room or zone with a rug and cozy chairs for greater feeling of hygge
- **Sounds:** favorite music or radio show or being away from a busy main street in another room of the home. Would earplugs or noise-canceling headphones be better to create quiet? Or could you try singing your favorite songs?
- **Smells:** scents from candles or perfumes, cooking, your pet, or freshly washed clothes
- **Textures:** fidget toys (sensory items that feel good to touch, such as squishy balls or PlayDoh), soft materials,

> warmth from a hot-water bottle, a weighted blanket, or natural materials, like pebbles, wood carving, and sand
> - **Taste:** Is there a familiar taste that feels calming or reminiscent of positive moments?

C for Connection

Since humans need to connect with one another for survival, our nervous systems are wired to develop close social bonds with others. Our green, social engagement enables this; moments of social connection when the hormone oxytocin is released make us feel calm, affectionate, and safe. Oxytocin also has restorative powers to help us heal from illness and injury. The neural networks involved with the social-engagement system are in areas of the body that even tiny babies can control early on in order to build the essential social bonds they need for survival. These include muscles of our faces and neck, eyes, voice, and ears, all of which have a modulating effect on heart rate. A baby's social-engagement systems help them to communicate and bond with their caregiver by:

- searching for eye contact
- making noises of pleasure (gurgling and cooing) or distress (crying)
- pulling happy or unhappy facial expressions
- distinguishing faces from other visual patterns in their environments and turning their heads toward them
- distinguishing human voices from other sounds and, again, turning their heads toward them

From the perspective of a helpless baby, the quality of the social bond with a primary caregiver, known as their attachment, is the main way of ensuring survival in a world where they have no independence. This means that a lack of engagement from their caregivers is interpreted as a threat. You can see this in videos of development psychologist Edward Tronick's still-face experiment in 2012, where the mother–infant interactions were observed. During this study, the mothers were instructed to stop responding to their child's attempts to interact with them by keeping a "poker face" and being nonresponsive to gestures like toys being offered to them by the youngster. The child became upset and, even after the mother stopped behaving in this way, there was a period of confused behaviors that indicated temporary disruption to their social bond: the child wanting to be close to her and reaching out but also averting her gaze.

If you were lucky enough to have primary caregivers who were attuned to your needs and able to regulate their own nervous systems, then this will have helped you to learn how to soothe your own nervous system after becoming upset or dysregulated. This leads to high vagal tone, meaning that your ventral vagal nerve is functioning at a level that enables you to cope well with stress (i.e., you can move up and down your gears smoothly). The good news is that low vagal tone can improve with self-soothing practices (which we get to in Chapter 5) and compassion (which we will cover in more detail in Part 3).

CO-REGULATION

An important way in which the social-engagement system supports us to feel safe is through co-regulation: the passing of messages between two people's nervous systems as to how safe or dangerous a situation is. When a child is upset, the calming presence of their parent, soothing and figuring out what they need, conveys an implicit message of safety to the child. This allows them to gently move back into green mode. A lot of parenting and caregiver support has this concept of co-regulation at its heart, encouraging adults to tend to their own nervous-system needs so they can meet the needs of their dependents.

Co-regulation continues to be important during adulthood as well. Notice how you feel when a colleague is rushed and anxious compared to being with someone who is steady and grounded. An important aspect of a therapist's work is to soothe their own nervous systems before starting a session to help them stay regulated in the face of their clients' distress—something that is very containing and healing. If you are in a human-services profession, then you will also be doing a lot of this work: essentially loaning out your nervous system to people who are dysregulated by things like injury, illness, and stress. Psychologists and therapists have regular supervision where they can get emotional support for this work, but this is not a regular feature of most jobs. I had a friend who used to work in a customer-facing role with highly distressed people who were about to lose their homes due to debt. She received no emotional support in this role at all and said it was never considered to be something that should be provided by management. But without appropriate support, long-term exposure to others' distress depletes us and co-regulation starts to go in the wrong direction. We catch their distress and feel worse rather than being able to offer a steadying presence. This is a common cause of a high level of burnout in human-services jobs.

BLOCKS TO CONNECTION IN MODERN LIFE

The strong urge for connection never leaves us and is one of the essential core needs in adulthood for helping us to stay regulated.

This is why we feel more relaxed when the body language of those around us is open and welcoming; why we glance at others' eyes for cues of kindness and warmth; and why we perceive that we have done something wrong when a voice becomes monotone or loud.

Our modern environment interrupts the cues for human connection. According to Gartner, a technology company providing research and advisory data to businesses, 40 percent of meetings were held online in 2020, set to rise to an estimated 75 percent in 2024. This coincides with increased reports of Zoom fatigue (exhaustion from overexposure to video-conferencing). Research into the reason for this highlights: overly intense eye contact when zoomed in on faces which feels threatening; having a constant image of oneself on screen (which we don't have in face-to-face interactions); and stress and anxiety from numerous data sources in the chat function and seeing multiple people at once. In group meetings, the clunkiness of the interactions, such as the stilted silences when you all fear you'll talk over one another, also interrupts the flow and sense of connection.

We are also logging on to social media more than ever to try to meet our innate need for connection, but here interactions are more about "likes" and "shares." Social media's "success" comes from its aggressive application of one type of psychology principle to hold our attention: behavioral reinforcement (that is, positively reinforcing behaviors that keep us on the platform in question). But our social interactions in the real world don't work like this. So not only do we find it hard to tear ourselves away, but it also triggers comparisonitis which is harmful for our mental health and prevents genuine connections.

Data from 2024 showing average usage per day from social media companies can lead us to estimate that the average person will spend about six years on social media in their life-time (assuming they start around age ten and continue until their early seventies). Not only is that time online getting in the way of connecting meaningfully with people who are actually present with us, but, in the words of Deb Dana, author of *Polyvagal Theory in Therapy*: "As we rely more on online conversations to communicate, there are fewer opportunities to exercise our social engagement circuitry."

Without practice, we can lose the confidence and skills for social connection. In January 2023, an article in *The New York Times* promoting a daily eight-minute phone call to friends and family to improve connection was followed by an exploration of this in *Stylist* magazine. They identified how low confidence was in many millennials when speaking on the phone, which, it turned out, was due to their self-perception of having a low level of skill in this through lack of practice.

We used to live in villages where we were nourished by a sense of belonging and had access to our elders' wisdom and a familiar, supportive community. Now, we may take on employment or pursue courses far from home and with colleagues in far-flung locations because transport is so accessible and online working is so advanced. The emphasis on choice and competition trickles down to everything from schooling and health to leisure activities. We can choose to travel further for our education and hobbies than ever before, but this has a knock-on adverse impact on our community cohesion.

Without proper human connection and opportunities for co-regulation, we become lonely. A 2022 survey by the UK Office of National Statistics showed that almost 50 percent of people in Britain feel lonely. Within the workplace, America's most lonely professions are: legal practice, medicine, science, engineering, and civil office. A physician who had left her profession due to burnout shared with me how isolating and lonely it had become, with the high-stress job being conducted almost exclusively alone rather than in a team, and an implicit message of failure if you needed to ask for a colleague's thoughts, let alone the idea of emotional support for something that has been intense.

Because human connection is so fundamental to our well-being, loneliness sets off our amber, protection mode. This is why loneliness is as much a risk factor for physical-health conditions as the more commonly recognized ones of obesity, smoking, and lack of exercise.

This is typically accompanied by worries about being "a burden," or that "others won't get it," and "I need to sort *myself* out." To overcome loneliness, we need to give our social-engagement system time to reconnect which takes some courage when we are feeling vulnerable and disconnected.

QUICK CONNECTION GLIMMERS

You can get connection glimmers from actually connecting with someone, but even imagining connection will stimulate the right neural networks and release oxytocin.

Two-minute option:

- Smile and say hello to the next person you see.
- Cuddle your pet (co-regulation doesn't just happen between humans; it can also occur between an owner and their pet).
- Look at videos of someone you feel affection for.
- Close your eyes and picture someone you care about (visualizations can stimulate the same neural networks

---

as actual experiences but this might take practice; see page 190 for more on this).

Ten-minute option:

- Listen to a familiar, conversational podcast.
- Call a friend or family member.
- Go out to sit on a bench where there are other people nearby (such as the park).

C for Choice

Without choice we lose our sense of agency and cannot uphold our boundaries or act in alignment with our values. This contributes to a feeling of being trapped or disempowered which, as we saw in Chapter 2, triggers our threat responses.

NOT ENOUGH CHOICE

For our nervous system to move fluidly through its gears we need freedom to choose actions that allow this. If our ability to choose is curtailed, we feel trapped and become more fearful.

In the present day, we are so bombarded by choice of anything from shampoo brands and cereals to mindfulness apps that it can be easy to miss how limited our choices are around the bigger life issues like work (such as a sabbatical or working part-time), parenting, money, and living standards.

Caregivers, for example, are often faced with very tough decisions due to limited choices, like whether to give up their job, home, or caring completely. In paid employment, options to take a break, such as an extended vacation or reducing workload by transferring to a role that involves fewer hours and responsibilities, are rarely financially possible when there are bills and mortgages to pay.

Reduced agency within work has been shown to increase stress and lead to employee burnout. Examples include micromanaging and enforcing top-down methods of carrying out tasks rather than allowing employees the freedom to carry out their work in the way they see fit. This reduction of choice leaves people feeling powerless and unable to uphold healthy boundaries, such as going home on time, working according to their values, and saying "no" to more work.

The other reason why we have curtailed choices is our own beliefs and the meanings we give to situations which come from not only messages about what is acceptable from our current situations but also our early life experiences. Beliefs that delegating means we've failed, that it is lazy to decline a project, and that we are letting our colleagues down if we don't do the overtime all reduce our perception of choice. We will come back to the sources of power that limit our choices (many of which are not obvious to us) in Chapter 7.

TOO MUCH CHOICE

A friend I visited when she was off work with stress asked me for my opinion on what she could do to feel better. She showed me the two mindfulness apps she'd subscribed to and placed an armful of self-help books on the table. She then struggled to remember which one she'd seen certain techniques in and seemed confused and overwhelmed about which to follow. An ironic example of modern life bombarding us with its superfluous choices. Too much choice means we have more decisions to make which is exhausting and interpreted as threatening by our nervous systems.

In a 2001 study in California, shopper behavior was observed around two displays of fruit jams. One had twenty-four jars and the other only had six. They found that 60 percent of people stopped at the more exciting display of twenty-four jars compared to only 40 percent who stopped to take in the smaller one. However, the buying behaviors showed the impact of too much choice on the ability to go through with a purchase, with 30 percent of shoppers from the small display going on to buy a jar compared to a tiny 3 percent from the larger display; the latter participants suffered from decision paralysis.

This research demonstrates that humans are attracted to choice, but too much of it pushes us into amber due to choice overload where we then feel stressed, avoidant of decisions, regretful, and demotivated. A clear example of how this plays out is in parental burnout where parents report being baffled by conflicting advice. There are many books on sleep, eating, sibling rivalry, and so on, but which do you choose, and how do you make sense of your child's tricky behaviors when a visitor or friend gives advice stemming from a different standpoint?

In *Motherwhelmed*, her book about parental burnout, Beth Berry gives examples of the tricky choices parents have to make on a daily basis, and, importantly, how draining this is because you never quite feel like you're getting it right. In choosing one option you are saying no to others that represent important values you hold; but it's impossible to adhere to those among all the other pressures. One example that Berry cites is: "Is it more important to keep the house clean or the kids engaged?" (Choosing between your value of orderliness and being present with your kids.)

QUICK CHOICE GLIMMERS

Two-minute option:

- **Remind Yourself You Have a Choice:** What can I move in my body right now that would feel good and responsive to a need I've not been paying attention to?

   Examples: Stand up and do a stretch; sit and roll your shoulders or push your arms into a stretch; walk into another room and take in the view from the window; run up and down the stairs a few times to refresh yourself; put on a favorite song and sing along.

- **Remove Too Many Choices:** What small action can I do next that would cut down the number of distractions and choices to help me feel better?

   Examples: If working on a computer, close all the tabs down that keep distracting you; put your phone in another room to improve connection with your kids or focus on your work; delete some apps that you don't use; unsubscribe from email newsletters for two minutes.

Ten-minute option (do this when you feel replenished, as decision-making is hardest when we are in amber and red):

- Do an audit of when you get stressed and see if this is related to decision-making. Can you make a plan to reduce this? For example, delete a subscription; put away the extra cereals and just leave two visible to choose from in the morning; lay out clothes the evening before.

Chapter 5

HOW TO SOOTHE YOUR NERVOUS SYSTEM INTO GREEN MODE

After being out sick with stress for two weeks, Sarah knew she couldn't go back to the same pace of work when she returned to her job. She also dreaded the backlog that would be waiting for her. Even engaging in therapy felt daunting, but the concept of glimmers seemed tolerable. She felt open to try recognizing these potential moments of calm or safety. Once she started to look for them, they began to appear. Whereas before, when she went into the break room where her colleagues were talking and headed straight to a quiet corner to do her grading, she now tried joining the conversation for a few moments first, experiencing a connection glimmer. She stopped to notice how much she enjoyed the peace that descended when the kids all left for their next class and took a two-minute opportunity to enjoy another glimmer with a gaze at the view of the playing fields from the window—a context glimmer. Although these small moments of anchoring in safety did not solve the stresses causing Sarah's burnout, she was allowing herself to lean into these glimmers and find some brief respite from her busyness. Then I introduced her to some tools for settling her nervous system.

When someone is stuck in a cycle of dysregulation, interrupting it is not be easy. If it was, they would have broken out of it already. Understanding how your nervous system works is empowering, but you also need to practice working with it. Repetition is what lays down the neural networks required for new habit formation. When you start something new, don't mistake the natural feeling of being challenged for a sign you're getting it wrong or that it doesn't work for you. This is normal; stick with it. New habits get easier over time because our brains are plastic: They are shaped by the things we do repeatedly.

When we are in amber or red modes we feel the physical intensity in our bodies and this leads to overthinking and excessive worrying. So when we soothe the body, it can communicate to the brain that the emergency is over, enabling our systems to regulate and thoughts to de-escalate. This is the principle behind the therapeutic tools in this chapter. Regular practice of these strategies when we are in green mode builds up the muscle memory ready to implement them effectively when we need to strategically regulate ourselves out of amber and red modes.

The tools you need in any moment will depend on whether you are mostly in red or mostly in amber mode. Discovering this involves listening to your body to recognize your own experience of being in either one (see the table on page 69 for help with this).

The following table looks at the main areas of the body for stimulating the ventral vagal nerve.

Area	How to Gently Activate This	Quick-Try Options
Mouth	Verbalizing sounds releases pent-up tension in the throat muscles and the vibrations around the mouth and throat activate the ventral vagal nerve.	Hum or sing one of your favorite songs.
Neck	Gently turning your head from side to side, up, down, or in circular motions moves the "curiosity muscle"—the sternocleidomastoid which runs from the back of the head down the neck to the top of the chest. Cold stimulation in this area has a regulating effect, too.	Look around the room and recite out loud (or in your head) all the things you can see that are blue. Get a cold flannel and place it on your neck. Play around with temperature; if you benefit from a very cold stimulation, put a wet flannel in a plastic bag in the freezer and take this out to use as necessary.
Eyes	Allowing your focus to broaden out to the wider space around you (the whole room). When we are in amber and red mode our pupils constrict and we have a more contracted view. When we broaden our focus to a more panoramic view, this can reduce stress and anxiety.	Look up and forward and relax your eyes so you can see as much of your environment and body as possible.
Lungs and Chest	Rhythmic and diaphragmatic breathing.	Breathing exercises (read on for these).
Ears	Listening to music or a calming human voice, especially a familiar, compassionate voice, will stimulate the inner ear muscles while the prosody is interpreted by our systems as a sign of safety.	Put together a playlist of five tunes that lift you up; save this under favorites and listen when you need it. Listen to an audio message from someone who cares about you.
Larger Muscle Groups	Movement will release pent-up energy stored in the muscle groups. Gentle stretches or yoga moves elongate the muscles and allow built-up tension to be released.	Learn three or four stretches (e.g., from yoga or Pilates and move through these gently; cross-crawl—explained later).
Heart	Breathing will regulate your heart rate. Warmth and imagining compassion to flow into your heart from external stimulation can be regulating.	Breathing exercises; place your hands over your heart and rest them there for a few minutes.

The next table shows how you can go about regulating your nervous system to come back to green mode.

Steps	Amber Mode	Red Mode
Step 1	Notice whether you are in amber or red mode.	
Step 2	Discharge the excess stress hormones to close the stress cycle.	Thaw out; bring energy back online.
Step 3	Ground yourself: Orient to the present moment and cues of safety in your current context.	
Step 4	Stimulate your ventral vagal nervous system to come back to green using breathing, soothing touch, tapping, or visualizations (see pages 98–108).	

STEP 1: NOTICE

Pause and scan your body from head to toe, mentally noting how each bit of you is feeling. Notice any sensations or numbness or tension—whether your heart beats quickly, whether your muscles are coiled for action, or whether you feel like crawling into bed right now. You can do this at any time in your day, but particularly good moments are the transition points when you move on to a new activity. The reason for this is twofold: first, it is a natural break which can help you to remember; second, different activities require different things from us—some require a slowing down to reflect, others a social connection, others high energy—and part of the problem in burnout is that these activities have all run into each other for too long and are all being carried out in one gear.

Some ideas for transition points are as follows:

- Finishing an item on your to-do list
- Before you start a meeting or videoconference
- Ending work for the day
- Heading out to get your kids from childcare

- Starting bedtime routine with your kids
- Sitting down to eat lunch or dinner
- Just before you get into bed

STEP 2: ENCOURAGE YOUR NERVOUS SYSTEM TO SHIFT OUT OF AMBER AND RED

We start with body-based exercises for you to move through.

Out of Amber: Discharge the Excess Stress Hormones and Energy
If you're finding it hard to pause long enough to do Step 1, this is a sign you are in amber mode. When you're in amber you feel rushed. You might be speed-reading this or skimming it while also fidgeting or tapping your foot. Your nervous system is telling you to run or attack. This is why it feels uncomfortable not to be on the move. You have an excess of adrenaline and cortisol that needs to be discharged before you can soothe yourself back to green mode.

The quickest way of discharging the excess hormones is to burn through them with movement. When you have a burst of intense activity, you naturally tire yourself. This then initiates the urge to rest which is what we are aiming for. There are also, however, options for when high-intensity movement is not possible or inappropriate, as shown in the next table.

Low Intensity	• Play with fidget toys. • Jiggle or shake your legs. • Bilateral taps (see page 105) on your knees or shoulders. • Tighten a group of muscles, such as your facial muscles or arms. Hold for a few moments then release. Repeat a few times. This is a brief version of a longer practice called progressive muscle relaxation (PMR, see page 107).

Medium Intensity	• Stand up and do some stretches. • Pace or walk around the room, up and down the stairs, or around the block. • Clean the windows, sweep, or vacuum. • Try a cross-crawl exercise (see page 106).
High Intensity	• Go for a jog. • Attend an exercise class. • Exercise at the gym. • Dance around the room. • Do star jumps or run up and down the stairs.

Out of Red: Thaw Out and Bring Your Energy Back Online

Feeling heavy, fatigued, and demotivated? In burnout, my clients report that this can be at its worst in the morning as they try to get going, during decision-making moments as they grapple with what to cook for dinner or which route to take, or when transitioning out of activities that they don't really want to stop doing, such as getting out of the shower, ending a coffee break, or telling the kids their screen time is over.

These heavy feelings are not your fault. It's not that you are lazy. They are signs of where your nervous system is at right now: in some state of freeze or shutdown. While the previously described movements in amber mode would also work here, they may require more energy than you feel you have and therefore be too much. Instead, you may need more gentle movement to bring energy back into your system. Start very slowly and build up speed as you begin to thaw and have more access to energy again.

The following are small movements that can help to thaw you out slowly:

- Moving your neck and head to slowly look around you, moving your eyes around the room, too.
- The self-hug: There are a few variations of this, so play around to

see what feels good. The first option is to place one hand under your armpit and wrap the other around your shoulder, so it feels snug. A second option is to place your hands around the tops of your arms and slowly rub them up and down as you might do when you feel cold and want to warm up. Make sure you stay with this for a few minutes (as long as it remains comfortable) to get the benefit.

- Swaying or rocking from one foot to another.
- Sitting on a swing or rocking chair (if you have one) and gently rocking back and forth.
- Chewing something crunchy, like a raw carrot.

STEP 3: GROUND YOURSELF

By orienting into the current environment, we can tune in to the cues of safety that are available and this helps us to find an anchor while we ride out the intensity of feelings and anxious thoughts.

Consider the following grounding strategies:

- Technique of 5, 4, 3, 2, 1: Notice five things around you that you can see, four things you can touch, three things you can hear, two things you can smell, and one thing you can taste.
- Bring your hands together and rub them, noticing the sensations of warmth and the feeling of touch.
- PMR can help orientate you to your body (see page 107).
- Cold water, ice, or flannel, particularly placed around the cheek and neck area where research shows it has the strongest impact on heart rate variability. Focus on the sensation of cold to ground yourself further.

STEP 4: SOOTHE BACK INTO GREEN MODE

After Steps 1 through 3 it should be easier to stimulate your ventral vagal nerve and bring yourself back into green mode. Some of the following techniques may feel very simple and involve repeating exercises you've already tried. If you are not accustomed to caring for yourself, you may get urges to stop initially; if you notice yourself becoming agitated due to this, go back and repeat Steps 2 through 4.

I'd recommend trying to come to terms with a soothing breathing practice. These are the quickest and most effective ways of sending messages of calm to your body because they engage the vagal brake (see the following).

Soothing Breathing Practices

The vagal brake is our hearts' pacemaker: the speeding up or slowing down of our heart rate according to what a situation requires of us. Heart rate is not only faster in amber mode (because this is a state of urgency—move quickly!) but also more erratic. The vagal brake brings the heart rate down again allowing a regular rhythm which, in turn, supports green mode to come back online.

So how can we actively *choose* to apply the vagal brake when our heart beats automatically without our conscious input? Fortunately, we have one internal bodily function that, though it acts automatically most of the time, can be brought under our conscious control, and this is breathing.

Controlling our breathing is the most effective method we have of applying the vagal brake. Slow, rhythmic breath slows the heart rate and gives us a more regular gap between heartbeats which improves the exchange of gasses coming in and out of the lungs (oxygen in and carbon dioxide out). This means we are getting rid of more waste matter which, in turn, improves the quality of blood being provided to the organs. With the right fueling, the brain starts to think more clearly, and all of this communicates to the body that we are now safe.

When a heart rate monitor is used to trace the heart rate of someone feeling stressed, the electrocardiogram (ECG) line looks like a jagged mountain range with tall peaks and low troughs, and the pattern is erratic. However, if you ask them to follow a soothing breathing practice for three minutes, the ECG line calms down to a gentle-looking wave. It becomes regular and less pointy, and the beats settle into a similar middling-range.[*]

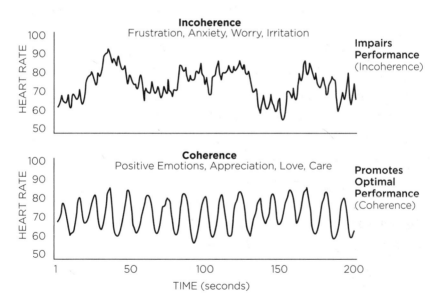

*Image courtesy of the HeartMath® Institute: www.heartmath.org.

You don't need to be experiencing a panic attack to have a heart-rate pattern that resembles the incoherent trace. Even mild stress can cause you to hold your breath or tense up in a way that causes erratic breathing.

I often recommend to my clients that they download a breathing biofeedback app to their phones when they first practice breathing exercises to keep themselves motivated. These biofeedback tools allow us to see what's happening inside our bodies and determine whether our efforts are working. These apps require access to the phone's camera and LED flash.

- **HeartMath:** This gives you a baseline score in your heart rhythm (called a "coherence score") and talks you through a breathing practice so you can see the real-time impact on your score. You can get a one-week free trial of "coherence training" (i.e., breathing practice which they recommend doing for five minutes a day).
- **The Self Compassion App:** This has a free biofeedback breathing tool with clear instructions and gentle music accompanying a three-minute practice. The app also includes a compassionate mind course (an extra paid-for resource which I highly recommend but is separate from the breathing tool).

THREE BREATHING EXERCISES

There are many breathing practices, and no one size fits all. It's a case of experimenting and finding one that feels comfortable but give it time. It might take a little while to get into it. If after experimenting you still find breathing practices difficult to implement, see the help box on page 102.

There are three main principles for getting the most out of a breathing practice:

1. Breathe in through the nose and out through your mouth if you can.
2. A slightly extended exhale compared to the inhale, as this is when you are exercising the vagal brake the most.
3. An even rhythm: Every cycle should be the same—so, in for three and out for five and repeat. Or in for four out for six and repeat.

- **Finger Breathing:** A simple method of counting the breaths. I like this one because you can practice it discreetly under a desk at work or college, and if you do both hands you will definitely have taken at least ten slow breaths by the end of it. Hold your left hand in front of you. Use the index finger on your right hand to trace along each finger, slowly breathing in as you trace up each one and exhaling as you trace down.

- **Diaphragmatic or Deep Belly Breathing:** Take a deep breath in now. Which part of the body moved the most? If it was your shoulders, then you aren't currently breathing from your diaphragm, which means that your breathing is shallow. The diaphragm is the stretch of cartilage below the lungs. When we breathe deeply, this should dip into the belly, giving the lungs more capacity to enlarge to allow plenty of space for oxygen and carbon dioxide to interchange with one another. As we age, we tend to hold more tension in our stomach muscles, which prevents this from happening.

  To deep belly breathe find somewhere to sit or lie and place one hand on your stomach and one on your chest. Imagine that there is a balloon inside you and you are gently expanding your belly to give the balloon space to enlarge. This gentle movement draws in the air at your nose, so the focus of attention is on the expansion of your belly rather than the intake of breath per se.

- **The Cyclic Sigh:** This is a relatively new breathing exercise by neuroscientist Jack L. Feldman, which a 2023 study showed to be one of the quickest ways of calming us when we are in amber or red mode. Neuroscientist Andrew Huberman, who was one of the study's authors, advocates using this exercise in real-time heightened stress, which means you can use it when you are about to do something very anxiety-provoking or stressful to help stabilize you enough to continue.

Breathe in through your nose. When your lungs feel comfortably full, take one final sip of air to top them up. Now slowly exhale through the mouth until your lungs have emptied again which dispels the maximum amount of waste matter (carbon dioxide). Repeat. It is recommended that you try to do this for five minutes, but that may be a goal to gradually work toward.

TROUBLESHOOTING COMMON OBSTACLES WITH BREATHING EXERCISES

- **Dizziness:** As you start to breathe more deeply, dizziness can be a side effect of the extra oxygen coming in. This is not dangerous, although you might find it more comfortable to sit or lie to do your practice.
- **They're Not Working:** To override the well-rehearsed physical response of amber and red modes, you will need to practice these exercises regularly, ideally more than once a day. To begin with, you might benefit from practicing when you are in green mode.
- **They're Making Me More Anxious:** If you aren't accustomed to tuning in to your body, you might experience some anxiety as you bring awareness to it and suddenly notice how tight your chest feels or how tense your muscles are. This isn't necessarily a sign that you have gotten worse. It's just a sign of what was already there but you are now noticing it. These issues should start to reduce with practice. Obviously, if you have breathing-related physical issues like asthma or chronic obstructive

---

pulmonary disease (COPD), a focus on the breath can be triggering and you might benefit from trying other options in this chapter instead.

- **Going Too Fast:** Due to the urgency in amber mode, it could be that you are simply breathing too fast to get the effects required. The counting should help with this, and you can add a word between each number—"one elephant, two elephant," and so on.

- **Zoning Out:** If you have experienced severe trauma in your past, it's possible that the slowing down resulting from the breathing goes too far and you end up in the red mode of shutdown. Some traumatic experiences have such a strong impact on the body that the survivor struggles to trust their body. Certain things can be triggering, such as breath work, particular poses, or touch. This can be worked through very gently, but you may benefit from extra support.

Soothing Hand Practices

Your hands are among the most soothing tools you have at your disposal after breathing exercises. When you place your hands on your skin, oxytocin is released. If you place your hands in areas where the ventral vagal nerves cluster, you also gain the additional benefit of gently stimulating these nerve clusters which adds to the soothing effect on your system. If you rub your hands together before you do these hand practices, it will make your hands nice and warm before you place them on your body.

It's best to try all of these, as you may find you prefer one over the others or like transitioning through them in a flow:

- Place both hands over your heart and rest them there for a few minutes. Apply enough pressure to feel comfortable. Play around with different amounts of pressure to see what feels good. Or you may prefer to hover your hands just a couple inches from your heart, tuning in to any sensations of heat in the air under your hands. Imagine compassion (warmth and kindness) flowing into your heart while you do this.

- Place one hand on your forehead and one on the back of your head at the base of your skull where the top of your neck is (the occiput). Rest them here until your raised arms feel too tired or swap the arms over if you wish. Again, you can close your eyes to help you focus in on the sensation.
- Place one hand on your forehead and one on your heart. Rest them here until your raised arm feels too tired.
- Place one hand on your heart and one on your stomach for as long as is comfortable and you start to feel the effects. You can also combine this with deep belly breathing (see page 101).
- Place one hand on your tailbone (the end of your spinal column that is central to the nervous system) and one on your occiput. Do this for as long as is comfortable and you start to feel the effects.

You can try adding a calming word or phrase to these hand postures. It's important to find soothing wording that feels acceptable; overly positive platitudes are unlikely to do this. Softening your tone of voice and the pacing of your words will further activate your green mode's social-engagement system. You might find it effective to use wording that you have heard in the past from someone who cares about you or that you've said to someone you care about. My four favorites are:

- "I'm doing my best."
- "This too shall pass."
- "This is not an emergency."
- "I'm safe."

Soothing Tapping Exercises

Bilateral stimulation is the activation of the left and right hemispheres of the brain in quick succession. We do this when we carry out an activity that uses the left and right sides of our bodies. You naturally engage in bilateral movement when you cycle, walk, jog, swim, or even knit.

Bilateral stimulation is utilized in an evidence-based therapy called Eye Movement Desensitization and Reprocessing (EMDR) through eye movements, taps, or beeps in your ears. EMDR is suitable for overcoming trauma and anxieties. The bilateral stimulation accelerates the capacity to process traumas (updating how traumatic memories are held in the nervous system).

Our eyes move back and forth as we move through the world. Research suggests that this bilateral activation dampens down the brain's threat response enough that we don't freeze up every time we encounter a potential threat. So we are alert enough to be wary but freed-up enough to approach the problem rather than back away from it.

HOW TO PRACTICE BILATERAL STIMULATION

There are a few options for this exercise. The simplest is to tap on your knees if you're sitting down; or, if standing up and trying to be discreet, you can put your hands in your pockets and gently tap the tops of your thighs.

A method we teach in EMDR therapy is called the butterfly hug: holding your hands out in front of you with your palms turned toward you, cross one in front of the other and hook your thumbs together. Now place your hands across your chest, so the tips of your fingers are around your collarbone. Now you can tap. One hand taps, then the other—not both at the same time.

When you are tapping to bring calm, I recommend a slow tap and then stopping if you don't feel good or if it's bringing up upsetting feelings or images. You can use "one-elephant, two-elephant" counting to pace yourself. Once you find a rhythm that feels soothing, you can stop repeating the words. Try this for one to three minutes.

TAPPING WITH A VISUALIZATION

In the same way that images of natural scenery can stimulate the nervous system as if you were physically there, images of certain people or animals who make you feel safe can stimulate it, too. You can develop a calming image by thinking of a place that is special to you. Common favorites are beaches, woodlands, being with a pet, or doing a form of feel-good exercise, like cycling, swimming, or dancing.

When you visualize your favorite scene, focus on what you can "see," as well as smells associated with this place, the sounds, and how it feels to move or "touch" things, such as sand, water, grass, or fur. Once you feel calmer, notice this feeling in your body and add in the slow bilateral taps. You need to practice this a few times when you are in green mode before trying to access it in red or amber.

Soothing Cross-Crawl

Cross-crawl exercises are any movements that involve crossing the midline of your body. This activates the left and right hemispheres of the brain which has the added benefit of bilateral stimulation; increasing the movement intensity helps discharge excess stress hormones. This exercise may not be advisable if you have high blood pressure or back issues. If this is the case, consult a doctor first.

Lift your left arm up, then raise your right knee and bring your left hand down to touch the knee. Repeat with the other side of your body. Continue with this until you feel that you've burned off some energy and are beginning to feel pleasantly tired.

Soothing Tense Muscles with Progressive Muscle Relaxation
When you tighten your muscles and hold and then relax, you set off a releasing of *all* the tension that they have built up with stress. Because your muscles are naturally relaxed when you are in green mode, the message communicated by your nervous system to your brain during PMR is that the danger has passed and it can return to a rest state.

Here's what to do:

- Find somewhere quiet to lie or sit where you won't be disturbed.
- Set the intention to stay focused on your body during this process. If your mind wanders off, gently guide it back to the muscles you are focused on. Take five slow, rhythmic breaths to help with this.
- When you tighten a muscle, focus on the sensation of tension and then the sensation of release.
- Work through these muscle groups, pausing for two to three slow breaths between each one:
  - Feet and toes (scrunch them up)
  - Calf muscles
  - Upper legs and glutes
  - Stomach muscles
  - Shoulders (squeeze together and up)
  - Arms and hands (create a fist and fold your arms into your body)
  - Face (scrunch your face)
- End with tensing your whole body up and allowing it to go limp.

A GIFT TO YOUR FUTURE SELF
At a time when you are feeling calm, a wonderful gift you can give to your future self is a "soothing bag" containing all

the tools you need to calm your system when overwhelmed. You could use an old glasses case or pencil case if you want something small and discreet when out and about or a box somewhere at home.

Here are some suggestions for what to put inside:

- The steps in this chapter are written down so you don't have to make decisions when you are struggling to think straight.
- A reminder of your favorite breathing, hand-soothing, and grounding exercises.
- Sensory items (see the box on page 80) that help your nervous system feel safe, such as calming photos or pictures, essences or oils (lavender or similar), a fidget toy, a plush toy, headphones, and a device for your playlist.
- Written-down coping statements that help to remind you that your nervous system is activated, that this situation will pass, and that you will be OK.

SIGNS YOU ARE STARTING TO COME BACK TO GREEN MODE

Your soothed green mode is more subtle than your red and amber modes. It can be hard to notice it, but if you are in green mode you are likely to find that words like *content, quiet, calm, still, resting, relaxed, peaceful, chilled, cozy, serene,* or *comfortable* resonate with the way you are feeling.

You might also feel more connected to your surroundings, and, if green follows a period of being in amber, your sense of urgency may begin to lessen. Alternatively, if you are coming into green after a period of being in red, you might feel your energy slowly picking up. As you start to get better access to your rational-brain functioning, like the ability to see alternative perspectives and problem-solve, the pace of your thoughts might also shift. Physically, you may yawn or notice your digestive system kicking back in with gurgling sounds in your stomach. Socially, you may feel more able to talk to others or to reach out for help.

What If I'm Not Coming Back into Green Mode?
The important thing to remember is that humans are complex; psychological tools like these aren't the equivalent of, say, tightening a bolt on a pipe so that the leak simply stops. Dysregulated nervous systems require persistent but gentle care and attention, and, over time, the movement between gears will become smoother and easier.

For this to happen, the practices I've covered here need to be repeated regularly. That's including when you are not dysregulated (i.e., when you are already in green mode, as this is the best way of getting started—much like exercising to develop stronger muscles). A daily practice using the ideas here will help you to access them more easily when you need to use them strategically.

An effective way of introducing these strategies into your routine is to habit-stack, adding your new habit to something you already do regularly. I practice four minutes of soothing breathing when I brew my morning coffee, for example.

Bear in mind that no two humans are the same. How you respond to these tools (or others) will be informed by your own past experiences as well as the current pressures you face. If you've suffered from severe childhood trauma, practices that focus on the body can be particularly tricky early on and you may benefit from more support.

WHEN TO GO DEEPER WITH BODY-BASED APPROACHES—AND HOW

If you find, despite these practices, that you remain numb or panicky, that zoning out isn't improving over time, or that you have unpleasant experiences you didn't expect, such as nausea, throat tightening, or pains in your body, these are signs that you are holding a lot of trauma in your body. This could be underneath your burnout, making you feel worse or making it hard to get better. We often see this in therapy. Someone will come for an issue such as burnout and with gentle exploration realize there's an underlying issue that wasn't apparent to them before.

There are forms of therapy that focus deeply on the body, releasing stuck bodily stored trauma and improving your vagal tone. The research into these therapies is still new, but there are studies showing promising results. I will cover other psychological therapies in Part 4, but if you think you would benefit from further body-based practices, here are a few options:

Trauma Release Exercise
This is a series of seven movements that encourage a deep muscle vibration to release stored tension, helping the nervous system to find balance. The exercises are led by a practitioner and feel pleasant and soothing. This can be carried out on a one-to-one basis or in group workshops.

Trauma-Informed Yoga
Regular yoga practice has been shown to have a stronger impact on anxiety than other exercise such as regular walking. Trauma-informed yoga includes the same moves as regular yoga, but the instructions are more invitational rather than direct. This gives you a chance to listen to your body and move it in a way that

feels good; it also improves your sense of choice which, as we've spoken about earlier (see page 87), is really important for returning to safety.

Somatic Experiencing®

This therapy focuses on noticing and responding to the sensations in your body and following a framework to help you release any trauma trapped there. There is emerging evidence that this can support people who meet mental-health diagnostic criteria in addition to building resilience (the ability to respond to stress in a healthy way).

Part 2

THE FORCES THAT DRIVE US TOWARD BURNOUT—AND HOW WE GET STUCK THERE

When working with clients presenting with burnout, we look for the experiences and beliefs that led to the coping behaviors associated with it, such as overworking or taking on too much responsibility. By becoming consciously aware of the forces that drive them toward these behaviors, it is possible for them to develop compassion for their overwhelmed nervous systems and become empowered to stick with the techniques to improve this—even when it's tough.

Beliefs are formed throughout life starting in childhood through messages received from the environment, such as culture, big-T and little-t traumas, and caregivers. In therapy, we tend to see a combination of external and internal pressures behind each case of burnout. Becoming aware of internal pressures and where they came from enables us to navigate away from unhealthy coping patterns that are contributing to burnout.

The information in Chapters 6 and 7 paves the way to putting it all together to create a road map out of burnout in Chapter 8.

Chapter 6

UNDERSTANDING PAST EXPERIENCES TO CONNECT THE DOTS

Suraj loved his job with the architect firm. Their ethos on sustainability was aligned with his own, and the projects excited him. He was still a junior but could see himself as a partner there one day, and this aspiration fueled him through the frequent late nights.

He knew he was sharper, calmer, and more efficient when he meditated in the morning, and he used time-blocking (dividing the day into blocks to focus on different tasks), which helped him to manage his workload, allowing time to go out for a lunchtime walk. And on days when things were going well, he would stick to this routine. But as soon as a customer asked for extra design revisions, or a colleague asked a favor, he felt unable to maintain his own priorities and rushed headlong into "doing mode" with everything feeling urgent until he had responded to all requests, which left him anxious about the outstanding tasks on his own agenda.

When we explored this together, he recognized how it was fueled by fears of not being good enough and letting people down. However, everyone at work said he was efficient and attentive. So why did he find it impossible to stick to his plans and let people wait a day? Why did he have to bust a gut to get stuff done for everyone else all the time?

HOW OUR EXPERIENCES INFLUENCE OUR INTERNAL PRESSURES

How we respond to everyday demands like emails, requests, and opportunities is informed, in part, by our early life experiences. Suraj grew up with parents who had high expectations for him and his career. They would be visibly disappointed when he didn't get top-of-class grades, so he worked hard to avoid displeasing them. Yet when he did achieve good outcomes, instead of receiving praise he was told not to show off, for fear of upsetting his less capable brother. He had therefore developed key fears that others are critical of him and that he is not good enough, which was fueling his perfectionist behaviors.

Our Beliefs

To navigate the world, we need to understand how it works and our place within it. As such our brains are meaning-making machines: these meanings (aka beliefs) revolve around ourselves, others, and the world. They inform our responses to the things that happen to us, the people around us, and our own thoughts and feelings.

We constantly absorb information from our environments and the events we experience, incorporating it and updating our preexisting beliefs accordingly. This allows us to function as best we can. Messages from the world might be made explicitly ("You let me down") or implicitly, from the way people around us behave or treat us. For example, if your parents never invited you to talk through friendship problems, the implicit message

116

was "people must deal with social problems on their own." This would lead to you having a belief in adulthood that prevents you from leaning into social support when you need it for fear of being seen as a burden or failure.

Our Bodies' Responses

Not only do experiences impact our beliefs, they also form memories. When people use the word "memory" they are often referring to the visual or narrative component of an event; this is called "explicit memory" and is only half of the story. Memory is also encoded in the body and our emotional brain in a way that we don't consciously choose to remember. This is known as "implicit memory." Positive implicit memories come from events that made you feel safe; say, the smell of favorite cookies being baked, the feel of having your hair stroked, the wallpaper in your grandparents' kitchen.

Implicit memories quickly inform the nervous system about whether or not a situation is safe. This type of learning is particularly strong in events that were aversive, like little-t or big-T traumas, because survival depends on the ability to quickly access memory about whether a current situation is similar to a previously threatening event (and therefore a risk).

In adulthood, we might notice implicit memories popping up when certain people, demands, or situations trigger a strong emotional reaction or coping patterns, and these can contribute to our burnout behavior. For example, perhaps you have set the intention many times to leave work at 6 p.m. but, when your boss raises an eyebrow as you pack up, you are reminded of those times your mother would tut and criticize you; you become tense and are still at your desk two hours later as a result.

In therapy, we explore personal experiences right back from the beginning because early life is particularly important in shaping our nervous-system responses and laying down important implicit memories.

Our Attachment Relationships

Attachment is the bond we have as babies with our primary caregivers; typically, parents, grandparents, or other adults closely involved with our upbringing.

Because babies constantly seek connection—their very survival is dependent on their caregivers' responsiveness—when they sense disconnection (through things like lack of eye contact, angry or blank facial expressions, or not being listened to or seen), it makes them feel unsafe and distressed.

Babies and young children require their primary caregiver to see their needs and respond to them appropriately, which both soothes them in the moment and teaches them to do this for themselves.

Infants cannot understand what need they have because they are so new to their bodies and experiences in the world. All they know is whether they feel OK or not OK. The caregiver has to figure out the baby's need before they can respond appropriately. This is a challenging job, and the way they respond depends on both their ability to attune and the prevailing parenting ideas at the time. Their ability to attune is also influenced by many factors, such as their mental health; preoccupations and worries about work, finances, and life events; use of drugs and alcohol; and their ability to tend to their own needs and soothe themselves.

The way your caregiver typically responded to your needs will have led you to develop a set of responses that optimized your chance of feeling safe with them. Being on the receiving end of frequent dismissive comments like "Don't be ridiculous, that's not worth crying over" may have led to coping responses designed to reduce feeling invalidated, such as avoiding crying in front of others or keeping quiet about negative events.

These relational patterns are called attachment styles and they inform how we interact with friends, colleagues, relatives, and partners in adulthood too. Those early cues of safety or danger in social relationships will inform how safe and trusting we feel of others and how we respond to them when they approach us or make demands of us. Ultimately, our nervous systems are looking to make connections with other humans to feel belonging, acceptance, and worthiness—all of which equate to feeling "safe." But insecure attachments can make this challenging, setting us up to watch for cues of danger, which, in turn, contribute to an accumulation of stress.

These patterns can cause us difficulties in our relationships with others, unless we are aware of them and know how to work with them, and they can also correlate with burnout. When we experience emotional pain, work is a handy device to hide behind—a distraction from the discomfort of feeling unseen, unworthy, rejected, or not good enough. Our attachment styles affect how well we can develop and maintain protective social connections with people around us, partners, relatives, and colleagues. Adults who have insecure attachment styles may also have access to fewer healthy skills in self-soothing. Feeling stressed may feel more familiar to them and, therefore, an acceptable state of affairs and not one worthy of intervention.

It is important to know that psychological interventions (such as those discussed in this book) can assist with unhelpful coping patterns related to attachment. Plus you can *earn* secure attachment as an adult through a process of self-discovery and insight into the reasons why you feel compelled to respond in certain ways. It is possible to learn new skills to self-soothe and foster healthy relationships with friends and partners in adulthood.

THE INSECURE ATTACHMENT STYLES

There are three insecure attachment styles. Take a look at the descriptions to see which resonates with you. You can also search online for the Adult Attachment Questionnaire if you'd like to get extra feedback about your own attachment style.

Dismissive and/or Avoidant

This pattern emerges when someone had caregivers who weren't consistent in meeting their needs, in particular dismissing or failing to see them—say, when the child searched for connection, none was forthcoming and they were left alone to deal with problems and strong emotions. Feeling ignored or rejected is familiar to them. Adults with this dominant attachment style tend to:

- notice that intimacy is accompanied by fear of being let down, and relationships are therefore kept at arm's length or at a surface level
- minimize or ignore their stress levels, pushing down these feelings and plowing on
- be more independent than others because self-sufficiency was a skill that developed early on; this can be a strength, but it can also make it hard to trust that others will be there for them without being let down
- have a strong tendency toward competitiveness (comparing self to others, monitoring progress, setting high standards, and so on)

What This Means for Burnout: If you recognize this attachment style in yourself, it's worth thinking about how you put the barriers up when you begin to feel close to someone. People with this attachment style are more likely to get overly involved in work at the expense of home life. I had a client who found his partner "suffocating" if they spent too much time together and felt more anxious on the weekends when this was likely to happen. On weekdays he worked late into the evening, and this was burning him out. Work was his escape from intimacy. Learning to befriend his emotions, connect to his values, and talk to his partner about his needs within the relationship were some essential steps for his recovery.

Unhealthy competitiveness often links back to experiences of being rejected or not noticed, leading to excessive striving behaviors, which compassion expert Paul Gilbert calls insecure striving; even in situations where someone *logically* knows they aren't inferior and are, in fact, very capable, fear of past inferiority can still trigger these competitive striving behaviors to avoid feeling that fear again. This behavioral pattern is exhausting and linked to higher rates of difficulties like anxiety and burnout than for those with secure non-striving behaviors.

The "Strive to Avoid Inferiority" scale is helpful for self-assessing insecure striving (see the Resources section on page 267).

Preoccupied and/or Anxious

Someone with this pattern likely had caregivers who struggled to meet their needs dependably, giving mixed messages about what was required of the child or being unable to be consistent with soothing them. Sometimes the caregiver was overprotective and other times they were overwhelmed themselves. The child picked up on their anxiety and was pulled into a role of looking after the caregiver. In adulthood this means that you may:

- be hyper-attuned to the needs of others and also feel responsible for them; this contributes to people-pleasing, which you do to reduce the possibility that people you care about will become distressed
- be hypervigilant or sensitive to problems and therefore often in a low-level state of alert, so that you are ready to respond quickly

- find it hard to sit with problems, making you hyperresponsive to them; this leads to more amber "fight" behaviors in the form of checking, reassurance-seeking, trying to fix problems quickly
- find it takes longer to recover from high-stress situations due to a dearth of soothing strategies and hypervigilance

What This Means for Burnout: Insecure striving is relevant in this attachment style, too. But whereas that fuels competitiveness in someone with an avoidant attachment style, in people with anxious attachment it is more likely to fuel people-pleasing: striving to keep others happy. People-pleasing is a key reason why burned-out individuals continue to say "yes" to demands, even when they have nothing left to give, and feel so guilty when they attempt to take essential downtime.

Often, people with this attachment style believe that their self-worth is dependent on how well they meet the needs of others and feel distressed if they cannot do this effectively. For example, Sandy was the eldest daughter to a very anxious mother. In therapy, we worked on her overinflated sense of responsibility for her siblings—for example, she would cook dinner most nights of the week for everyone in the house (all adults), often catering to their food preferences, too.

People with this attachment style are more likely to be juggling many plates—their own projects, as well as noticing (and absorbing) everyone's feelings, which adds to emotional exhaustion, then preempting what they'll need and often sacrificing their own time and energy to meet these needs. It can feel very difficult to put boundaries in place because they feel responsible for managing the negative emotions of those around them if they say "no." In fact, for some people "no" is not just a tricky word, but one that makes them feel so unsafe that it's almost impossible to say it.

Fearful and/or Disorganized

Children of caregivers who were frequently scary, confusing, abusive, or inconsistent may have a propensity toward a disorganized attachment style. They had to cope alone with emotional abuse and neglect or inconsistent behaviors from their parents and learned to deal with their strong emotions independently. This can continue into adulthood with potentially chaotic or highly avoidant strategies for negative emotions and a strong fear of rejection and abandonment. There is heightened sensitivity to others' emotions due to overexposure to traumatic experiences, and they are more likely to misread facial expressions as signs of being rejected or criticized and therefore believe they've upset someone when they haven't or that others are angry with them when they're not. Due to all this, there can be ambivalence in their actions; for example, reaching out to others for connection but then feeling overwhelmed and fearful when they start to feel close and so withdrawing again.

What This Means for Burnout: An important additional fear in this attachment style is that of being abandoned, which fuels behaviors designed to avoid this, like working hard, people-pleasing, and trying to prove one's worth, whether through achievements or external proof like promotions and certificates. Unfortunately, getting closer to someone doesn't tend to feel soothing for someone with this dominant attachment style; instead, it can result in more fears of getting hurt, so there is often a pattern of striving to get closer to others, then reacting with fear when this happens. In addition, there may be a struggle to cope with high-stress situations using healthy habits because these weren't taught in childhood. In fact, they may even believe they're not worthy of self-care or the care of others because they didn't receive this in childhood. This closes down the possibility of letting on how bad they feel, while asking for support seems almost out of the question. There is also a higher chance that a person with this style of attachment learned to emotionally detach from intense emotions.

There are strategies associated with this attachment style that, while effective in the moment for getting through difficulties, do not align with long-term personal goals, such as use of substances, shopping, doomscrolling, and self-harm. These are often quite impulsive reactions to intense emotions or stress that leave someone feeling disappointed with themselves. This can create in them a vicious loop of low self-esteem, because these behaviors are often followed by self-critical thoughts, which make them feel worse, and when they feel worse they feel emotional pain, which they then avoid through more unhealthy avoidance strategies.

THE SECURE ATTACHMENT STYLE

This develops when someone had a caregiver who generally noticed and met their needs enough that they internalized a message of being safe and accepted. This allowed the child to connect with their feelings and learn to respond to them appropriately.

If you have a secure attachment pattern in adulthood you are:

- able to feel worthy of others' affection
- able to feel soothed by others when they try to comfort you
- more likely to have appropriate boundaries with others
- able to lean on friends/partner when you need support, while also able to tolerate their distress when they then lean on you

At a nervous-system level this form of attachment gives your ventral vagal circuitry the best start in life, where the attuned nature of the caregiver's attention allows down-regulation of distress, which trains the child's nervous system to move fluidly through its gears (linking to higher vagal tone). This makes stress in adulthood more manageable for them and healthy soothing options come more easily.

What This Means for Burnout: People with secure attachment can still feel burned out but they might find it easier to engage with self-help strategies earlier on or reach out for help. All humans, no matter their attachment style, have an innate wish to achieve and are motivated toward resources that secure safety; in a modern-day context, this is social status and money, both of which we get from our studies and work. But in secure attachment, there is generally less fear of failure, and secure non-strivers are able to feel accepted whether or not they achieve certain outcomes.

MESSAGES THAT INFLUENCE OUR PROPENSITY TO BURN OUT

Attachment styles are not the only influence on someone's relationship with work. During therapy with a client, we also spend time considering the implicit messages that we pick up from our surroundings, such as how others behave and what they pay attention to—all of which feed into our beliefs and implicit memories. Here are some common examples (although this is not an exhaustive list).

Work Messages

Anything that our caregivers modeled, praised, or showed attention to was very important to us in the early years of life, and we are more likely to do more of these things in an unconscious bid for their affection. For many people I work with, there was strong modeling of overworking and parents who praised their children when they followed suit—the importance of work often being placed above other things. Take Sheena, whose mother returned to work in a busy legal job only three days after giving birth to her. She remembers her mother being agitated in the evenings when she was trying to get back to her laptop after putting her to bed and having meals interrupted with work calls. The message was: Work is more important than anything else. This is a message that often permeates school, as well as home, with school rankings centering on exam grades and not on pupils' holistic well-being.

An overemphasis on work means losing the nervous-system benefits that children get from playing, which can protect from burnout. Play gives children opportunities to practice transitioning from amber to green mode. When I played "tag" with my three-year-old, she would find it exhilarating up to a point, then suddenly cry out for me to stop chasing her, as the energy of her amber mode suddenly tipped into a feeling of threat rather than fun. This would be met by a hug and comforting words that she was OK, helping her to regulate back to green mode, and strengthening her vagal tone (essential to resilience in the face of toxic stress).

Success Messages

Noah came to therapy due to lack of motivation, strongly fearing failure. He told me a memory of standing in front of his parents with a grade he thought he could be proud of (98 percent) and being asked, "What happened to the other 2 percent?" He had many more stories like this, so the message was very clear: Anything less than perfection is a fail.

There are two main motivations for achieving: growth-seeking and validation-seeking. The first is linked to expanding one's knowledge and skills. The second is a pressurized place of feeling second best and needing to prove oneself. This concept originated in 1998 with researcher and psychology professor Benjamin Dykman who explained that the validation-seeking achievement is a consequence of critical parenting, where perfection is overemphasized. Achievement is therefore a threat-based response and can make it hard to tune in to one's need for rest and recuperation because of not feeling safe enough to actually do this.

This idea was added to a few years later by psychologist Carol Dweck who introduced us to fixed and growth mindsets. A fixed mindset means that success is measured by the outcome, where, for many, only an A or 100 percent will do. This makes us fearful of criticism and challenges because the trial-and-error that is part of the process of learning is interpreted as failure. A growth mindset, on the other hand, is one that praises the *process* of learning, such as trying new things, persisting in the face of setbacks, and viewing mistakes compassionately as part of the journey. Many people in my clinic who overwork and find it hard to stop striving grew up in homes where fixed mind-set was the norm, often feeling they were only as good as their last achievement. This traps us in burnout behaviors and exhausts us.

Family-Rule Messages
There are often implicit rules in the family around how difficult emotions or events are talked about (or not), who the head of the family is, and how everyone treats each other. Here are some general categories to consider:

- Fun is allowed *or* fun is not allowed.
- Putting yourself first is selfish, so you mustn't have boundaries *or* putting yourself first is healthy.
- Don't show emotions or talk about them *or* it's OK to have all the emotions—we can work through them together.
- You must be good and perfect *or* you can be whoever you are.

We can carry these rules with us into adulthood and feel guilty or uneasy if we act in a way that is not aligned with them. If you grew up in a family that made it hard to have boundaries, do relaxing activities, or feel joy, then you will be more vulnerable to burning out.

OUR PLACE IN THE FAMILY

Birth order impacts the way people treat us and the availability of resources, like our caregivers' time, energy, and finances. The following examples are broad trends, mostly from Western research, and therefore don't represent all families:

- **Firstborn:** Research shows that the eldest is often praised for supporting their younger siblings and is expected to be more responsible at a younger age. They often bear the brunt of their parents' hopes and expectations and are more likely to conform to these and try to please them. In my therapy work, I see a common trend where an eldest child is likely to be high achieving and conscientious, step into leadership roles, and be listened to within the family. In the workplace, roles that reflect these qualities (managers, caring jobs, or those with a lot of responsibility) are particularly at high risk for burnout.
- **Subsequent Children:** Middle children have fewer expectations of responsibility placed upon them and, as a result, tend to feel more liberated to follow their own paths. Some younger siblings may feel that they are compared to their older siblings and are walking in their shadows, which can either feel demotivating or have the opposite effect of making them want to prove themselves. Youngest children are often seen as the "cute" ones and can struggle to be taken seriously, even as they grow up, which can make them want to prove themselves, too.

Things like birth order, your personality, strengths, and (perceived) weaknesses can lead to labels being assigned to you, and many families tend to do this. In my family I was the "sensible one," my middle sister was the "sensitive one," and my brother was the "funny one." The problem with these labels is that they trap us and prevent people from noticing our many other virtues. They can also get stuck as we grow up, in terms of both how our families see us and how we internalize them and believe this is how we must be. These labels then become the expectations we set for ourselves and what we use to measure our success in the things we do. This is something else to consider when looking at your own burnout backstory.

Family Social-Status Messages

Any prejudice that your family experienced as you grew up, due to race, sexuality, disability, religion, and so on, will have led to stress and threat responses in your caregivers that impacted their parenting, as well as shaping your own beliefs about your place and sense of belonging in the world. For example, someone I once worked with told me how her parents would frequently remind her that she had to work twice as hard at school as her white peers because doors wouldn't open as easily for her. Experiences of prejudice can range from overt discrimination to the less-easy-to-spot implicit biases and microaggressions (which can include micro-insults, micro-invalidations, and micro-assaults). Being looked down on by others can lead to striving behaviors in a bid to belong or prove yourself; they also chip away at your self-esteem over time.

Losses and Life-Gap Messages

Losses in childhood can include people and pets who were close to us. This can be from death, illness, or injury (your own or family members'), family separation, estrangement, or moving to a new area. Where someone played an important role in meeting our core needs the loss will be felt even more keenly. For example, a parent, nanny, or grandparent leaving may feel very upsetting and confusing and be experienced as abandonment if they were closely involved in care. Equally, a family pet dying can be particularly hard for the child whose bed the pet slept on every night, their warmth providing the comfort required to fall asleep.

"Life gaps" refer to periods in our lives where our hope and expectation didn't meet reality. For example, if you were thrown into a caring role for a family member during your teen years, you would have missed the socializing and studying that others of your age enjoyed and that you had anticipated for yourself. Life gaps carry a strong sense of loss and grief.

All of this is painful, and humans are good at safeguarding against future pains (often subconsciously). One way of safeguarding is to try to control as many aspects of a situation as possible. For example, in the case of the young caregiver, they may overprotect and take on too much for their loved ones in a bid to ensure that further harm cannot come to them.

Another important aspect of losses in childhood is that we will witness how our caregivers cope with the emotional pain. In the past, it was frequently frowned upon to openly show grief or suffering, so I often find that my overworked clients witnessed their caregivers escaping into work or using busyness to avoid feeling their grief.

Messages Created by Bullying
Bullying, discrimination, and harassment can have a lasting impact no matter how old we are when they happen. It might be physical or emotional bullying, or trolling, and it could take place in person or online, and it is more likely to occur when there is a lower acceptance of diversity or when compassion is not valued

or emphasized by the local community or school. It can make us feel ostracized from the group—that we don't belong or have something inherently wrong with us. Our ability to cope with bullying is influenced by how much support we have from our peers, caregivers, and teachers. Verbally processing what has happened allows us to gain alternative perspectives that help us to distance ourselves from unhelpful thoughts that it's all down to who we are and that we are unacceptable.

Experiences of bullying can cause us to want to prove ourselves and protect ourselves from the possibility of being bullied again in the future by achieving high status.

Messages Transmitted via Parenting Norms

There are a few approaches to child-rearing with different emphases on how caregivers should discipline and support emotional and cognitive development. Dominant parenting styles change from decade to decade. The emphasis these days is on emotional development and learning to regulate emotions. But back in the day when you were growing up, you may have experienced a parenting trend that prioritized academic achievement or the idea that children should be seen and not heard. This means that, even if you had well-intentioned caregivers, you were likely to be sent to your room alone when you showed strong negative emotions, giving the message that intense emotions were not acceptable and that you had to learn to deal with these alone. That core need of connection was then withheld, contingent on being "good" rather than being available when needed to soothe back into green mode.

One result of overemphasizing external markers of success (academic or sporting achievements, for example) is the feeling that rest has to be earned rather than used as a tool for regulating and pacing yourself.

Chapter 7

THE EXTERNAL PRESSURES PUSHING US TOWARD BURNOUT

Anika's promotion to ward manager had come at a stressful time in her personal life with her father being unwell and needing daily support from her and her brother. So she was already overloaded before stepping into work where the new position involved constant firefighting of issues beyond her control, like finding enough staff to meet the minimum requirements. The team spirit and community on the unit had dissipated over the last few years after long-term staff members had left and vacancies hadn't been filled. Anika was convinced that the stress of working with so few resources and emotional support had led to higher incidence of staff sickness and faster turnover. It added to the feeling of being taken for granted; at least when there were regular team members on shift they could be attuned to one another and shown appreciation for their efforts. It was important in a role like this where the patients were feeling too poorly to do so, and higher management often overlooked this as well.

SIX RISK FACTORS FOR BURNOUT

Research carried out by social psychologist and professor Christina Maslach's team in workplace settings found six consistent external pressures that contribute to burnout. These pressures can show up in informal or unpaid settings too—at home and in community groups.

Overload

Too much to do and not enough time to do it is the most obvious reason for burnout, and the one with the strongest links to exhaustion—and it is not only employees who struggle with this. Parents, students, caregivers, academics, athletes, and self-employed people feel just as frequently that the expectations placed upon them are too much to manage.

Lack of Control

Having little or no agency over decisions about how you spend your time generates the feeling that you lack control—if you are allocated a project you don't want to work on, for example, or the future direction of an organization is changed by a merger. Many employers focus heavily on meeting targets to get funding or satisfy shareholders which leads to the micromanagement of staff.

Lack of control outside formal work environments includes similar situations, like having to fit in with others' plans or expectations, feeling you have few decision-making powers in your family, romantic relationship, or friendship group, or feeling that you are living in a chaotic environment.

Insufficient Rewards

Roles that entail monotonous work are unrewarding because they're boring, while those involving a long delay in seeing the finished project, or where you are only a tiny cog in a process, leave you feeling that you're not valued. Caring roles, including parents involved with the regular care of dependents, may not generate much gratitude or praise, and the value of what's being provided may not be fully comprehended.

We feel rewarded when we are involved in things we are passionate about, when we see the positive outcome of our efforts—such as the finished project—or when others recognize our efforts by showing us appreciation and praise.

Breakdown in Community

When we don't have a supportive community of colleagues, peers, managers, or family around us, we feel isolated and miss chances to co-regulate and be playful, both of which reduce our stress. The community also creates opportunities for someone to spot signs that you are overworking and rally round to prevent this from getting worse. A compassionate community is one that feels psychologically safe and one in which we feel able to speak up about things we feel unhappy about, both of which are very important for getting our needs met.

Lack of Fairness

If we see inequality or witness some people being treated better in a workplace, we feel angry. If we cannot voice this anger or it is invalidated, this leads us to become cynical about what we are doing.

Conflict in Values

Being asked to do things we don't agree with creates a mismatch in our values. This can leave us constantly feeling torn in two directions and drain us. For example, when I worked as a psychologist in the NHS, I wanted to spend a good amount of time preparing for client therapy sessions. But I also wanted to be considered a "good employee," which meant hitting the target of seeing a specific number of clients each week. These two values conflicted and caused constant tension for me.

Why Are These Six Factors So Prevalent?

There are many influences in current environment and culture that create downward pressure on our organizations, communities, and, therefore, us. Some of these are not very visible to us. They are also oppressive. Moreover, it is very hard for us to challenge things we cannot see. As a result we internalize messages from these oppressive influences, and they often shape the negative mindsets that are an important feature of burnout.

PRESSURES STEMMING FROM OUR CULTURAL NARRATIVES

Narratives are the ways in which certain concepts are generally spoken about and therefore understood to be "true," and dominant narratives in our culture create oppression that we may not be conscious of. Two ideologies that underpin many narratives in the West linked to burnout are patriarchy and neoliberalism.

Patriarchy is the idea that men should be in charge. This creates stereotypes about men and women that adversely affect both genders because they pigeonhole what is considered acceptable in terms of behavior, emotional responses, and roles for everyone.

Neoliberalism—the concept that prosperity hinges on individuals being self-sufficient and autonomous and, importantly, that too much regulation hampers this—has contributed to an emphasis on creating market competition, capitalism (social practices designed to accumulate wealth), and consumerism (the emphasis on the consumption of goods), all which have become woven into the fabric of our everyday lives. These ideals have contributed to why we feel like rebels or failures when we do things that go against the status quo (like resting or choosing not to buy the newest iPhone) and why we are so closely monitored in terms of our productivity (targets and values that align with output).

These narratives influence social policies, how our society and organizations are structured, and our relationship with work and rest, and then they are reinforced in marketing messages.

A dominant gender-stereotyped narrative that predates COVID-19 but which was intensified during that period is that nursing staff are "superheroes" or "angels." An article in the *Journal of Nursing Scholarship* considered the impact of this narrative on aspects of nursing, such as their work conditions, explaining that "providing a safe working environment is unconsciously less of a priority for people who have this super power to overcome adversity and whatever is thrown at them." It is no wonder that 62 percent of nursing staff report burnout if their essential needs are unconsciously being downgraded to "nice-to-haves."

This narrative not only impacts how politicians and hospital bosses create safe workplace environments but it also influences the meaning nurses make of their experiences at work. I worked with a nurse a few years ago who came to me believing she was a failure and not cut out for the profession. When we explored this together, we could see that she had internalized the unrealistic expectations implicit in the "superhero" narrative, inadvertently using it to guide her reaction to feeling worn out by workload and lack of agency. She wasn't a failure. She was in need of more rest, more staff to support her and her patients, more advance notice of her rota, better staff quarters to take a break. All of which are reasonable human needs that this narrative obscured.

The following are some more oppressive narratives that have come up in my therapy conversations with people experiencing burnout:

- **Work as Only Worthwhile If We Are Passionate About It:** In the book *Can't Even,* writer and journalist Anne Helen Petersen gives examples of how the language of "love" and "passion" has been woven in with work in recent years. She shows how destructive this idea is, effectively giving businesses the green light to create poorly paid but exciting-sounding jobs or unpaid internships. This, of course, loads extra financial stress on top of preexisting student debt and increases the chance that someone has to hold down multiple jobs at once (one to pay the bills and one that follows their true "calling" and so on). All ingredients for chronic stress.
- **Work as Only Being of Social Value If It Is Paid:** This makes a lot of invisible hard labor easy to dismiss as a contributing factor in burnout, such as caring for dependents, housework, do-it-yourself projects, emotional support, and studying.
- **White Races Are Superior to Others:** This influences the implicit biases and responses to people in marginalized groups, not only in the workplace but in all aspects of living. Professor Kenneth V. Hardy (from the couple and family therapy department of Drexel University in Pennsylvania) explains that the trauma of racial oppression (such as being persistently overlooked for promotions and judged negatively) leads to *internalized devaluation* (i.e., individuals feel incapable and less worthy). This, combined with the affronts of racial discrimination, contributes to lower-paid roles, fewer choices, impaired self-esteem, and overworking to compensate, all of which increase the risk of burnout.
- **Men as Providers:** This can cause significant distress to males when they cannot provide for their families. They are more likely to suffer from self-blaming ideas of failure if they cannot step into this role. This lends itself to insecure striving: attempts to achieve or to maintain social status and financial success. This narrative also denies men the space to voice their worries or concerns about work or career progression because this might

be construed as a weakness. One entrepreneur I worked with recognized how much harder he pushed himself in the lead-up to the birth of his second child; he regretted how little time he was spending with his family but felt compelled to provide for them. His burnout was a culmination of this and having no one to talk to about his disconnection from family and the effect it had on his sense of belonging to them.

- **Women as Nurturers:** This creates a sense that women are naturally meant for caregiving roles and may, in a similar vein to the nurses' experience (see page 136), reduce access to emotional support or acknowledgment that they may not wish to do these roles or that they find them laborious. In their book, *Burnout*, the Nagoski sisters link this to the concept of human-giver syndrome: the idea that society expects women in particular to give themselves in the service of others.

- **Millennials as Snowflakes:** The term "snowflake" is a relatively new and pejorative way of describing someone as overly emotional, overprotected, and unable to cope with opposing views. It is a narrative that has been particularly applied to the millennial generation and is damaging because it silences people when they try to stand up for their rights or make reasonable requests—like asking for a pay rise—which may protect from burning out. This group of people matured into the workforce during one of the trickiest financial periods in recent history, the 2008 crash, when workplaces were trying to make savings, so narratives that made it harder to ask for better pay and conditions would have benefited companies trying to make cuts and savings at the time.

HOW THESE NARRATIVES CONTRIBUTE TO BURNOUT

We internalize the aforementioned narratives as truth rather than one version of how life could be, and we unwittingly adopt them as guiding principles and standards by which we measure ourselves in our personal and work lives. The expectations of these internalized narratives make us feel stressed and reduce the control we have over aspects of our lives because we are being guided by external influences rather than our own desires and needs.

Negative Thoughts

Unfortunately, the unconscious oppression from these narratives shows up in our thoughts, causing negative mindsets (also known as our inner critic) in a way that makes it hard to spot and discount. This is why challenging negative mindsets can feel like an uphill battle—because the people and organizations around us unwittingly buy into these narratives as well and thus perpetuate them. For example, I worked with a mother to challenge her unhelpful mindset that she always needed to drop everything immediately when her teenage kids made a request. Therapy supported her to have healthy boundaries and to explore the benefits of this for her children who were learning to stand on their own two feet as well as being on the receiving end of a far less irritable mother. But she would often bring experiences to therapy of being put down by her own parents for drawing these boundaries, and she felt at odds with how her parent friends talked about doing things.

HOW CAN WE PUSH BACK?

The good news is that shining a light on how narratives put pressure on us empowers us to challenge them by responding with compassion and sensitivity to our distress. One compassionate response is to rest when we are overloaded. With all this in mind we could also consider rest as an act of rebellion against the cultural pull to always be producing, consuming, and in competition with each other. Compassion and rebellion all while we sleep, read, or watch TV!

The following table gives examples of ways in which we internalize narratives into negative thoughts, and I'll come back to tools for managing these thoughts in Chapter 11.

Thoughts We Have That Show How We've Internalized Oppression	The Narrative This Thought Is Linked To	Understandable Threat Responses That Lead Us Deeper into Burnout
Why can't I manage when everyone else seems to?	Self-sufficiency is very important. **This is important because:** It stops you asking for help and stops people talking about their issues for fear of looking weak.	• Withdrawal from others • An overfocusing on self-improvement • Not asking for help (especially in environments where the people you might talk to could judge you or you are in direct competition with, like work) • Ignoring signs of stress and trying harder to fit in with others
Other moms, dads, caregivers, teachers, nurses, insert-your-profession-here are doing it better than me.	We are in competition with each other and need to be the best to succeed. Competition is emphasized in capitalism. **This is important because:** It makes us feel threatened by others in the same position as ourselves.	• Insecure striving behaviors • Loss of self-confidence

I'm a failure because I don't go on nice vacations, don't own a house, or don't have a long-term relationship.	Success relates to your ability to contribute to the economy and buying power (required for consumerism to thrive). **This is important because:** It gives no appreciation for other aspects of life that are valuable in noneconomic ways and good for our well-being, like feeling connected, enjoying hobbies, feeling safe, or relaxing.	• Working harder to prove self and trying to reach high standards
I can't tell anyone how I feel because I don't want to burden them.	Individuals should be self-sufficient, and distress is a sign of failure. **This is important because:** It prevents valuable connection and devalues communities.	• Avoiding talking to others • Withdrawal • Worrying alone

Competitiveness

The financial and emotional pressure on people of all ages to "keep up with the Joneses," own the latest iPhone, or meet top-down targets set by management makes us feel insecure and encourages us to monitor our own and others' performances.

According to Social Comparison Theory (the idea that we have a primitive drive to compare ourselves to others in order to gauge our self-worth), this is natural to a degree. We assess our self-worth and value by comparing ourselves with others—something that our ancestors needed to do to ensure their safety within their social group with higher social ranking protecting them from being ostracized from the group. This leads to a natural tendency toward competitiveness, but it can be adversely affected by the outlined narratives.

Situational factors that skew this natural comparison process include having a lot of people to compare yourself to and an awareness of how close you are to the higher ranks (i.e., being closer to number one increases competitiveness). A few years ago, I worked with a financial consultant who told me about the weekly email he and his associates received in which their individual business figures were published and ranked from best to worst—an example of the competitive landscape being controlled for business purposes, putting high pressure on employees to avoid the humiliation of being at the bottom and creating a culture of overwork.

Some environments lend themselves easily to making social comparisons. For example, when we were in school, grades were a quick comparison tool, while in adulthood, certain work environments have staff bandings or hierarchies which are similar. But there are many situations—say, among our friends or neighbors—where there is not a quick comparison tool, and this is where busyness has stepped in to fill this gap. Boasts, such as "I've barely sat down all day," are our unconscious bid to secure our self-worth and ensure we rank highly among others, because busyness means we are producing and therefore of high social value. Sadly, of course, this busyness also keeps us separate, stopping us from pausing to connect and seeing how little this truly adds to our satisfaction in life.

There is one more painful twist in social comparison that is unique to burnout. Upward comparison (the process of comparing ourselves to people who are in a higher social position than ourselves) has the ability to be inspirational and motivational. But burned-out individuals are more likely to interpret this type of comparison negatively, feeling more inadequate as a result. Downward comparison (when we compare ourselves to those who haven't reached the same level of achievement yet) is also interpreted more negatively when we are burned out. It makes us feel worse because it triggers the belief that we are deteriorating and messing up. A classic example that most people relate to is how bad social media makes us feel—when we aren't in a good place, we often turn to scrolling to cope with our strong emotions or escape stress, yet this is where we are bombarded by images that encourage social comparison at a time when we are most likely to take negative meaning from it.

Our environments encourage competitiveness which adds significantly to stress while reducing our access to resources—compassionate connection with others, emotional support, and practical resources that we may feel weak taking up.

This has a ripple effect into our wider communities. For example, parents living in dense populations—where there is more competition for school placement—are exposed to more competitive talk at school about things like reading levels and school enrollment (e.g., public, charter, or private).

COLLECTIVE TRAUMAS IN THE WORLD
THAT ADD TO OUR BURNOUT

Collective traumas in recent years have left their mark on us, even if we aren't always thinking about them consciously. COVID-19, the climate crisis, warring countries, political turmoil, and violence against specific groups have built a traumatic and destabilizing backdrop against which we've attempted to live our lives. These events have made us feel afraid for our safety or more generally uncertain and, therefore, anxious, hopeless about change or about our futures, and angry at our leaders and perpetrators of violence.

We have all been touched by these issues, either directly or indirectly. They impact the decision-makers whose choices affect every one of us. They filter down to how our organizations act to "safeguard" for the future, often resulting in cuts, increased surveillance, or more rigidity in their procedures and policies. We can be left feeling like we are firefighting rather than progressing.

All this reduces our sense of control which, as discussed in Chapter 4, destabilizes our foundation of safety—the very feeling our nervous systems are striving for. Some think deeply about these world issues and are weighed down heavily by them, and there are small ways to manage this, and we will look at these in Chapter 11.

But before we look at that, we are going to develop the charts you need to find your way out of burnout.

Chapter 8

NAVIGATING AWAY FROM BURNOUT

After eighteen months of running his own company, Scott was finding it tough. The business was doing well, but this meant the workload was increasing and so were the pressures, yet he had nobody else to share the big decisions with or to lend him some moral support. Having given up the safety net of paid employment, he didn't feel he could turn down new opportunities, and now he was spending all his time and energy on his business as a result.

In the back of his mind, he *knew* he had options. He could take a day out to do his quarterly planning or set aside time to employ someone new, but he struggled to take actions like these. He would create space in his calendar for reflection and planning but then ignore the reminders. He was busy advising clients to make decisions that made sense for them. Why couldn't he make decisions or take actions to improve his own situation?

The truth was that those reflective spaces made him feel anxious. Pausing from the busyness of work simply allowed the unpleasant thoughts and feelings to make themselves known more loudly:

Thoughts:	Worries about looking foolish or being criticized if his business doesn't succeed
	Self-critical thoughts that he should be able to cope with all of this by himself and that getting support would equate to failure
	Beliefs that delegating could lead to a drop in standards and not knowing how he'd cope with this
Body Sensations:	Tension and knotty muscles, feeling fidgety, and a sense of urgency in his body, making it hard to sit still
Emotions:	Guilt and anxiety

HOW TO IDENTIFY YOUR OWN INTERNAL PRESSURES

In therapy, we look out for these types of negative thoughts, feelings, and emotions that are internal pressures driving someone on. We use what we find to formulate their pathway to feeling better.

Becoming familiar with your internal pressures is not only helpful on the pathway back from burnout but also provides empowering self-knowledge for keeping your working practices as healthy as possible in the face of external pressures (which you may have less control and influence over).

To map out internal pressures, we start by looking at the negative events in our pasts that have shaped our beliefs and reactions. This is an exercise used in CFT—a psychotherapy that improves your relationship with yourself through increasing feelings of inner safety and self-compassion; it helps us to understand how our pasts have created feelings of threat and strategies for coping that aided us through difficult times *then* but have unintended consequences or "side effects" that contribute to burnout *now*.

We start by considering life experiences like the ones I outlined in Chapter 6, from family, school, relationships, and culture to work, illnesses, and significant life events, like losses or moving (the first column in the following chart). From there, we can start to piece together the impact of these experiences. In what way did they inform our key fears? (These tend to fall into two types: fears about how others will treat or view us and fears about our internal experiences, like negative emotions or body sensations.) The second column of the chart refers to external and internal fears.

With these fears comes the urge to ensure they don't come true or to avoid them from happening again, which is why we tend to develop coping strategies in childhood to protect ourselves (the third column of the chart). The strategies that worked well for us at the time are often the same ones we use in adulthood. Some *may* still work now, but pausing to consider whether they are still the best option makes sense, because in adulthood we are likely to have more choices available to us and newer experiences to draw on for alternative ways of coping. What is more, our old protective strategies are often the key to understanding why we struggle to stick with the things that could help now, like self-care, setting boundaries, implementing more realistic standards, and so on.

With every action there is a consequence. Some might be intended—for example, if you get reassurance when you seek it, you might feel less anxious in the short-term. However, there can be consequences that we do *not* intend and that, in fact, cause us a whole new set of problems—perhaps your reassurance-seeking feels too much for someone else who backs off from the relationship, bringing it to an end. Or perhaps a consequence of getting projects done to a perfect standard is that you get asked to do more and then feel taken for granted.

Chart of Your Internal Pressures[*]

Life Experiences	Key Fears	Protective Strategies	Unintended Consequences
Life experiences and key events that led to internal reactions about yourself, others, and the world. Some helpful areas to consider:	What meaning have you taken from your life experiences?	How do you try to prevent your key fears from manifesting?	Protective strategies might help in the short-term but what are the longer-term unwanted side effects?
Family (e.g., conflicts, pressures on the family, attachment style, loss, rules, role in family) **Community and Culture** (e.g., stigmas or strong ideas in your culture that have an impact on you)	**External Fears** What do you worry about in terms of how others will treat you or think of you? Common fears are being rejected, abandoned, excluded, let down, harmed, or shamed.	**External Protective Strategies** What do you do to prevent your fears about how others perceive and could behave toward you? Common examples are self-reliance, people-pleasing, hypervigilance, appease, or reassurance seeking.	**External Unintended Consequences** How do your external ways of coping impact your relationships and the way others think and feel about you? Common examples include needs not being recognized by others, relationships lacking depth, feeling insecure, becoming socially marginalized, or being taken for granted.
School (e.g., academic and friendship experiences or bullying) **Relationships** (e.g., experiences that shaped your trust in others, belonging and responsibility) **Career** (e.g., experiences of being valued, given responsibility, listened to, etc.)	**Internal Fears** What do you worry about in terms of who you are and how capable or worthy you are? Common internal fears are about not being good enough, being weak or vulnerable, or being alone.	**Internal Protective Strategies** What do you do to avoid your fears about yourself from being realized? Common examples are avoiding or suppressing your own needs or emotions or being critical of yourself.	**Internal Unintended Consequences** What side effects do your protective strategies have on your thoughts, feelings, and body? **How do you relate to yourself?** How do your protective strategies affect your relationship with yourself (e.g., critical, dismissing, resenting). **Mood** What impact does all of this have on your mood?

*A CFT formulation by Paul Gilbert © 2022. Formulation template used with permission of Taylor & Francis through PLSclear.

Some of the unintended consequences can make us feel worse, setting off our key fears again which creates a feedback loop, and this is when we feel trapped.

The three most common protective strategies I see contributing to burnout in my practice are: perfectionism, people-pleasing, and avoiding strong emotions. Let's take a look at each of these in turn, but keep in mind that you may relate to more than one.

The Internal Pressure of Perfectionism

Perfectionism ranges on a spectrum from a harmless sense of diligence at one end to an unsustainable focus on getting things "just so," even to your own detriment, at the other. If you feel joy and pride in meeting your high standards and are able to pace yourself and take a break when you reach a goal, then this is likely to be at the healthy end of the spectrum. But if you don't often identify with those positive feelings and feel like you rarely get things to the standard you hope for, you probably sit at the more insidious end of perfectionism where it is taking its toll on your well-being.

There are three types of perfectionist, the first two of which are associated more strongly with burnout:

- **Rigid Perfectionist:** someone who seeks a flawless outcome because their self-worth feels dependent on it
- **Self-Critical Perfectionist:** someone overly critical of feedback who strives for perfection due to a belief that others expect this from them
- **Narcissistic Perfectionist:** someone who demands perfection from others

If you want to see which of these perfectionism styles you relate to most, you can self-assess using the Big Three Perfectionism Scale which is freely available by searching online. Here is Suraj's chart—he is someone whose self-critical perfectionism is adding to his burnout.

SURAJ'S CHART

SURAJ'S LIFE EXPERIENCES

Family

Successful professional parents who placed heavy emphasis on Suraj doing well in exams. Expected him to get As and a first-class degree. They weren't in the habit of praising him.

Competition was inadvertently reinforced between him and his brother.

His role in the family was the "golden child" or the one who was expected to do well.

Identified with the avoidant attachment style the most.

School Years

Enjoyed getting good grades, finding this rewarding. But was bullied for being nerdy. Suraj moved to different schools multiple times due to his dad's work relocating. He found it hard to adapt to new school rules and policies and tried to be as "good" as possible to avoid breaking them.

Sometimes he and his brother were the only children of color in the school (and local area), so people would stare and make him feel awkward. He stopped attempting to have close friendships due to the effort of trying to get past the feeling of being different and to avoid the disappointment when he transferred to a different school again. He coped with loneliness by throwing himself into academia, as this was simpler than trying to work friendships out.

Career

Had to work hard to get good grades in the competitive architecture field. Had experiences of being embarrassed by a tutor at work who didn't like his ideas. Endured high-pressure environment at work with unrealistic expectations, elevated standards, and regular sharing of targets around the office—who was hitting them and who wasn't.

SURAJ'S KEY FEARS

External

- Being criticized
- Being seen as not as good as others
- Being let down
- Being unable to trust others to be there for him

Internal

- Thinking he's not good enough
- Feeling insecure
- Feeling lonely

SURAJ'S PROTECTIVE STRATEGIES

External

- Following rules rigidly
- Plan, plan, planning
- Spending a long time perfecting work to a high standard
- Keeping others at arm's length
- Competing with others

Internal

- Doing everything himself, so he knows it's done to the right standard
- Setting high standards
- Sense of self-worth hinging on achievements
- Self-critical
- Exercising stringent self-control

THE UNINTENDED CONSEQUENCES FOR SURAJ

From External Strategies

- Procrastination (hesitation with starting something until he knows it will be perfect)
- Feeling isolated and not part of the group or team
- Everything he does takes longer than others (perfectionist strategies are time-consuming)
- Other interests are pushed out because they don't help with the goal of getting to the top of the career ladder

From Internal Strategies

- Disappointment with his achievements
- Low self-worth on occasions when he doesn't achieve what he'd hoped to
- Exhausted, as he finds it hard to rest

How He Relates to Himself

- Hard on himself when he "misses" a standard or loosens his self-control

Mood

- Feels low and anxious

The Internal Pressure of People-Pleasing

Doing kind things for others is not in itself a bad thing, but people-pleasing is not the same. It is insecure striving: feeling compelled to do things for others, even if it's at odds with your own wishes or values. It comes from an avoidance of threat, often from low self-esteem or feeling like you'd be letting people down or at risk of being ostracized if you didn't do it. Emma Reed Turrell, author of *Please Yourself: How to Stop People-Pleasing and Transform the Way You Live*, suggests there are four classifications of people-pleasing:

- **The Classic People-Pleaser:** Someone who takes pride in their ability to excel at putting others first and almost feels defined by it, their self-esteem being based on whether others feel good.
- **The Shadow People-Pleaser:** Someone who simply believes that others are more important than themselves; they might quietly people-please without making a big deal about it.
- **The Pacifier People-Pleaser:** Someone who fears any displeasure in others, so placates everyone, pushing aside their own feelings to avoid rocking the boat.
- **The Resistor People-Pleaser:** Someone who may not identify with being a people-pleaser because they don't engage in many of the behaviors, but only because they feel so concerned about how they'll be perceived or rejected that they avoid people altogether or grace them with their absence.

Here is Anika's chart; she is someone who identifies with classic people-pleasing.

ANIKA'S CHART

ANIKA'S LIFE EXPERIENCES

Family

Anika had an emotional and anxious mom and rarely saw her dad, who coped by working and avoiding home.

Putting her own needs first was considered selfish.

Her role in the family was to be the peacekeeper and to ensure her younger sister had what she needed and wouldn't upset her mom when she was having a bad day.

Identified more with anxious attachment style.

School Years

Enjoyed school well enough. Had a central role in her friendship group—was always the one to organize outings

---

and think of everyone's needs. Loved getting feedback from teachers about being helpful and conscientious.

Career

Gravitated toward a caring role and has always been surrounded by others who have normalized excessive giving to others. Had an anxious manager in her first qualified position who tried to micromanage her and the staff. Anika's heightened awareness of this anxiety set up a pattern among colleagues that fitted with her friendship groups growing up: fearful of displeasing others or seeing them stressed and overcompensating.

ANIKA'S KEY FEARS

External

- Being abandoned
- Being rejected
- Being humiliated
- Being seen as selfish

Internal

- She'll let others down if she doesn't take responsibility for them.
- She's not good enough.
- Her feelings aren't important; she shouldn't tune in to them.
- Being a burden to others would mean she has failed.

ANIKA'S PROTECTIVE STRATEGIES

External

- Never setting boundaries with others
- Trying to tune in to and anticipate the needs of others
- Pleasing others so they don't reject or criticize
- Checking she hasn't upset others (rereads texts)
- Always selfless

- Avoiding asking for help
- Trying to protect others from emotional upset
- Withdrawing from people who could offer moral support

Internal
- Taking all the blame when things go wrong
- Hinging self-worth on her ability to be of service to others
- Hiding or avoiding feeling frustration or anger at others
- Ignoring work–life boundaries

THE UNINTENDED CONSEQUENCES FOR ANIKA

From External Strategies
- Empathy-distress fatigue
- Finds it hard to accept support or care from others
- Feels taken for granted by others
- Feels worn down by everyone's needs
- Carries a lot of emotional weight from everyone's needs
- Is lonely

From Internal Strategies
- Not attuned to her own needs and body
- Dwelling on interactions
- Feeling guilty or anxious when at rest
- Is exhausted

How She Relates to Herself
- Critical of herself when feeling frustration or anger
- Blaming herself if others are unhappy

Mood
- Feels low or anxious when she self-blames

The Internal Pressure of Avoiding Strong Emotions

We all have emotions as a normal part of the human experience. They are helpful and important in ways that we will explore in the next chapter. It's natural to find negative emotions intense and to wish to avoid these, but some people struggle with this more than others. For example, some children grow up in families where emotions are communicated in an uncontrollable way, such as very angry or aggressive parents or a parent who cries a lot or who is visibly very anxious. Or the opposite, where emotions are never communicated or expressed, and this in itself gives the message that they shouldn't feel and that, if they do, it's a sign of a problem (for example, they're overly emotional, weak, or irrational). If this occurs, then avoidance of emotions through the distraction of work and aiming to protect yourself by getting a high-status role can be a natural consequence.

Here is Scott's chart—he is someone who identifies with avoiding strong emotions.

SCOTT'S CHART

SCOTT'S LIFE EXPERIENCES

Family

Scott's parents separated when he was young with his dad leaving them with no financial support. His mother was often agitated or impatient with him and the only grandparent in his life seemed to blame him for his parents' relationship ending. When Scott got upset or annoyed, his mother would tell him he was like his father, which was an insult because his father had been emotionally abusive and abandoned them.

School Years

At school, Scott sailed through with ease and particularly excelled in athletics. His coach encouraged hard work and

---

Scott became quite competitive. With all the school work and sports, there was little time left for friends, so he didn't develop any close friendships.

Career

Scott wanted to provide for himself and his mother, so he made it his aim to earn enough to do this as soon as possible. He became financially stable quite quickly but, in doing so, turned into a workaholic. After burning out in his corporate job he decided to set up his own business, which his mom disparaged.

SCOTT'S KEY FEARS
External
- Being abandoned
- Being rejected
- Being humiliated
- Being criticized or let down
- The unpredictable or scary emotions of others

Internal
- Doesn't feel acceptable as he is
- Doesn't feel good enough
- Feels his negative emotions are not acceptable
- If showing emotion, he might become like his father who abandoned him
- Needs to maintain an identity as capable and as a provider

SCOTT'S PROTECTIVE STRATEGIES
External
- Keeping others at arm's length so he doesn't need to show emotion or manage theirs

- Being independent and never asking for help
- Failing to delegate, doing it all himself
- Using work as an avoidance or to gain control, especially work that doesn't involve emotions

Internal
- Striving to succeed
- Suppressing emotions (trying not to feel)
- Withdrawing from people when feeling emotional
- Intellectualizing and staying with cognitive reasoning rather than listening to his body and emotions

THE UNINTENDED CONSEQUENCES FOR SCOTT
From External Strategies
- Lonely
- Feel worn down from doing everything himself
- Carrying a lot of weight of expectation to provide for others

From Internal Strategies
- Being unattuned to his body and emotions means he doesn't recognize how stressed he is
- Suppressed feelings bounce back in other ways: either coming back more strongly or via somatic issues (aches and pains or health conditions linked to stress)

How He Relates to Himself
- Hard on himself when emotions come to the surface, telling himself he's failed

Mood
- Feeling low or anxious when criticizing himself

The questions in the table on page 148 and information from Chapters 6 and 7 can be used to map your own internal pressures. Sometimes this can trigger your inner critic and make you give up which can make it an emotionally challenging exercise. To help you manage this, try imagining you are writing and reflecting on the life experiences of a dear friend rather than your own.

Part 3

REBALANCING TO RECOVER FROM BURNOUT

By the end of this section, you will have the concepts and tools you need to come back to balance from burnout.

Chapter 9

RESTORING BALANCE

Sarah (the burned-out teacher) had charted her internal pressures with me. As a youngster, she was expected to take on a lot of responsibility, caring for her younger siblings when her mom had bouts of depression and took to her bed for days on end. When her mom roused herself out of these episodes, she would often be critical of how Sarah had overseen certain tasks, seeming to forget that Sarah was still just a kid herself. Sarah therefore developed key fears that others were critical of her and that nothing she did was good enough. She compensated for this by trying to avoid others becoming distressed, anticipating their needs and stepping in quickly when she thought they might need something. At school, this meant she would often agree to extra playground duties or running an after-school club for an absent teacher rather than allowing the school to cancel it. In an environment that was chronically under-resourced and where demands were potentially endless, this had run her into the ground.

As her burnout progressed, she'd started to cope with the excessive demands by withdrawing. If she saw fewer people, she wouldn't need to absorb their distress and workload. But this also had a negative consequence where her colleagues couldn't see how much she was struggling and failed to offer help. Sarah felt alone and even more disconnected from the main part of the work she enjoyed: her team.

In therapy, Sarah started to slow herself down during the transitions in her day, so it felt less like she was chaotically running from one activity to the next. In moments when she felt flooded by stress and anxiety, such as at night if she woke in a panic or when the principal announced he'd be popping by for an observation, she had started to place her hands on her heart, take ten slow breaths, and remind herself that this feeling would pass (her favorite affirmation). This would soothe her in the moment, but she still found herself caving in during those excruciating silences in staff meetings when the head asked for a volunteer for something. She felt unable to resist the compulsion to help. Not offering felt lazy and selfish, which she found deeply uncomfortable. She wanted to know what she could do to break the habit and stem at least some of the flow of demands she was juggling.

Sarah was struggling with self-compassion. Her threat mode was activated when she considered asking for help or putting in a boundary around her time so she could have a break. This triggered key fears that others would think she was selfish and judge her. After all, that was what her mom had always done.

Sarah is not alone in struggling to tend to herself with self-compassion. People with unhealthy levels of perfectionism, people-pleasing tendencies, or difficulties tolerating emotions often find self-compassion hard or fail to see the value in it. A study in 2016 discovered that people who struggle to show themselves self-compassion tend to be high in care*giving* toward others yet low in care-*seeking* for themselves. Self-compassion actually requires the capacity for *both of these things*: giving ourselves care and being able to receive that same care *from ourselves*.

To help Sarah develop a healthy relationship with the demands in her life (and therefore recover from burnout), we needed another chart. This time we mapped her emotion systems, drawing on Paul Gilbert's "Three Systems of Emotions Regulation" used in CFT. According to this model, emotions have evolutionary roots, having developed to allow humans to survive in the world. Each of our emotional reactions occurs to guide our behavior according to important underlying motivations such as to care for one another (caring motivations) and to gain access to important finite resources like food, status, and social support (competitive motivations).

Here's how our emotions support this: Anxiety alerts us to possible danger, so we will get a strong urge to flee; anger flares up when someone has crossed a boundary, motivating us to reinforce it; sadness prompts us to seek out social support after a loss; joy occurs when we do things that are good for us in the long-term, like playing and socializing (the good feelings encourage us to seek out these moments again).

We can't help our initial emotional reactions. These hardwired responses might have helped our ancestors survive and thrive, but now these responses may be less relevant to us. An example is the flare of annoyance I get if I leave my chair during a meeting to go to the bathroom and then return to find someone else sitting in it— this is an old territorial reaction flaring up, even though my more evolved, rational brain can reason that I can sit in a different chair.

This means that some emotional responses clearly make sense to us given the situation, but sometimes we can be baffled by our reactions because they don't appear to fit. This is when they may have come from an older place.

Self-compassionate behavior involves listening to the wisdom of our emotions and then pausing to work out if the particular emotional reaction is warranted for the current situation before making a decision about how to behave.

The three-system model classifies our primary emotions into three overarching systems to thrive:

- **Threat System—Anger, Anxiety, Disgust:** Our threat system creates the emotions of fear, anger, or disgust, and these intense experiences prompt us to take immediate action to get to safety when we feel endangered. The type of action we then take to find safety is determined by which mode we are in (amber or red), and that, in turn, is dependent on the level of threat and our ability to find safety.

- **Drive System—Drive, Excitement, Vitality:** The drive system is associated with positive feelings, like enthusiasm, energy, and focus, that keep us on task and in pursuit of goals—feelings that incentivize us toward the resources we need to thrive, like food, social status, and reproductive opportunities. It's the buzz we get when we know we are on track for getting a promotion, when the person we like reciprocates, or when our favorite meal is placed in front of us. Our drive system maps on to the non-protection amber mode—the sympathetic nervous system energy we get when we are not feeling threatened.

- **Soothing System—Content, Safe, Soothed:** Humans need to rest and spend time bonding with social groups to build up strong connections they can rely on. This means being able to calm down enough to take a break and recuperate and nurture social bonds by giving and receiving care to and from others. This is vital for reenergizing after the heavy calorie-consumption of the other two systems. In this system, we feel safe and contented, and oxytocin is released. This maps on to the green ventral vagal circuitry.

MODEL A—IN BALANCE

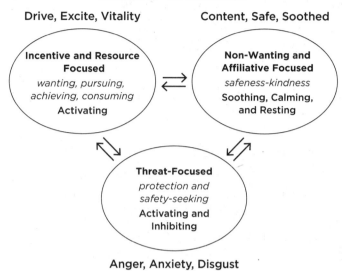

Drive, Excite, Vitality   Content, Safe, Soothed

Incentive and Resource Focused
wanting, pursuing, achieving, consuming
Activating

Non-Wanting and Affiliative Focused
safeness-kindness
Soothing, Calming, and Resting

Threat-Focused
protection and safety-seeking
Activating and Inhibiting

Anger, Anxiety, Disgust

MODEL B—OUT OF BALANCE

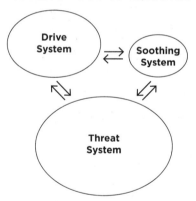

Drive System

Soothing System

Threat System

Model A shows the three overarching systems in balance, with the drive, soothe, and threat focuses all equal in size.* Model B shows the common imbalance when internal pressures contribute to burnout.

---

*Both models are adapted from Paul Gilbert, *The Compassionate Mind*, 2009, reprinted with permission of Little, Brown Book Group through PLSclear.

Overactive Threat System

Sarah's threat system—the system that veers us into red and amber modes—had become overactive. This was clear from her irritability, constant worrying, and the way she tensed up whenever the principal walked into the break room.

Our threat systems have a tendency to become more sensitive the more they are set off. This heightened threat response would have been a helpful survival mechanism for our ancestors. It makes our threat system hyperresponsive, a bit like a car alarm being set off when there is just high wind rather than a burglar. For Sarah, the pressure of the escalating demands of her job, with its increased targets and extra grading combined with an uncompassionate principal, was putting her threat system on high alert.

Overactive Drive System

The second system identified as overactive in the lead-up to Sarah's burnout was her drive system, the one that stimulates amber mode's passion, excitement, and goal-chasing zone (rather than its running, fighting, and survival behaviors). Drive is highly regarded in Western culture. We celebrate hard work and goal-driven behaviors. Add to this messages from early life around the value of success, perfection, and achievement, and it's easy to see why our drive systems become overinflated and can fuel our competitive mentalities.

The drive system can be used to dampen down an activated threat system. For example, Suraj was driven to overdeliver on his architectural projects to protect himself from feeling criticized or a failure, thereby dampening down his threat response. Sarah would take on the work of others on top of her own to avoid letting them down, thereby ensuring her status as a helpful person and avoiding criticism from her colleagues. The difficulty with an overactive drive system being fueled by a competitive mentality is that it can be hard to take your foot off the gas. You need to keep working hard to maintain your social status and rank because there's a fear that something bad will happen if you don't—such as being seen as a failure.

Keeping your foot on the gas means remaining on high alert for ways to succeed and therefore in "doing mode," too. But if you're excessively tuned in to how you're coming across and looking for the next way to prove yourself, you are far less likely to tune in to the stress signals in your body.

Understimulated Soothing System

A final emotional imbalance in Sarah's burnout was an under-stimulated soothing system (active when we are in green mode, our ventral vagal and social-engagement circuitry). This system had not been nurtured or valued much in her life which meant she hadn't established good resting, recuperating, and soothing activities for herself, and she also found it hard to receive care from others.

The dominant message in our society is that rest is lazy or a sign of weakness and "doing nothing" is a waste of time. To develop a strong soothing system, it helps to have witnessed people around you valuing self-care and connection and to have been on the receiving end of this soothing. This develops vagal tone and your ability to recognize dysregulation. If this was scarce in your life—and still is—the good news is that this is a skill that can be practiced and improved at any age thanks to neuroplasticity (the ability of the brain to establish changes through repetition).

HOW TO RESTORE BALANCE

There's a misconception that self-compassion can make us weak or that self-criticism motivates us to work harder, but, in fact, the science shows the opposite to be true. Self-compassion improves our ability to regulate our nervous systems and therefore to cope with stress. It strengthens our capacity to pick ourselves up after setbacks and reach our longer-term goals.

When our nervous systems are being overwhelmed, intense emotions can hog the limelight and internal pressures can fuel our inner critics. Self-compassion brings balance back, responding to our stress with kindness, understanding, and a wish to make things better. Self-compassion is more than the soothing system. It entails listening to the wisdom of *all* our emotions when they have something to say, then working out the most effective action plan rather than responding with a knee-jerk reaction. It entails regulating and soothing the nervous system using the methods in Chapter 5 and also learning new ways to respond differently to our inner critics or worrisome thoughts. It also entails prioritizing well-being.

Changing Your Direction of Travel Away from Burnout
Whether you identify with perfectionism, people-pleasing, avoidance of emotions, or all three, if you are in burnout you are likely to be using your drive system to dampen down threats, which means you are moving clockwise through the three emotional systems. When we move from threat to drive system rather than threat to soothing system before moving into drive, we run up against a few problems:

- You have less access to your frontal-lobe functions, such as creative thoughts and the ability to problem-solve and rationalize, which are hampered during amber and red modes.

- You are disconnected from your positive motivations for being driven, such as a wish to be a good role model or to share your knowledge and have shared experiences with people you care about. Instead, you are motivated by fears like avoiding criticism, rejection, or being left out.
- Last but not least, you are more likely to act with urgency and later regret actions that were impulsive, such as starting a project that hasn't been properly planned out or responding rashly to an upsetting email, adding stress and friction to your day.

By introducing tools for self-soothing, such as those we looked at in Chapter 5 (see pages 98–108), you essentially change the direction of travel around the three systems. But to support this anticlockwise journey, you also need to work on any blocks hindering access to your compassionate self.

TRAVEL COUNTERCLOCKWISE TO REBALANCE

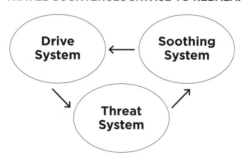

WHAT COULD BE BLOCKING ACCESS TO
YOUR COMPASSIONATE SELF?

Here are three common struggles where our compassionate self is concerned. You may find that all three are relatable or that one needs more work than the others.

You're Not Tuned In to Your Feelings
This means that you don't notice them. You engage in perfectionism, people-pleasing, and busyness-to-avoid before realizing what's brought you down this well-worn path. Perhaps you ignore or override intense emotions?

Your Inner Critic Is in Charge
You feel the feelings but don't have the skills to respond differently. You *are* able to notice your emotions and know that you need alternatives to people-pleasing, perfectionism, and avoidance, but your inner critic (which leads you to these patterns) is so demanding that it is hindering your ability to do anything differently.

You're Disconnected from the Compassion of Others
You don't let others in and find it hard to either ask for help or receive it when it's offered. Instead, you tend to try to solve all your difficulties on your own and hide when you are struggling.

The next three chapters will show you how to unblock each of these struggles and access your compassionate self.

Chapter 10

LEARNING HOW TO TUNE IN TO YOUR FEELINGS

Suraj was aware of how irritable he could be in the evenings with his partner. In fact, the increase in their arguments was the reason he'd finally decided to reach out for support; his partner had insisted this couldn't continue or he'd walk out. When we discussed emotions, Suraj looked at me blankly. He seemed only to identify with anxiety, and even this was only when it escalated into panic. During our conversation, he started to realize just how often low-level anxiety was present during his working day. But it was also more complicated than that. Sometimes there was sadness (for example, when his efforts went unnoticed) or anger in the form of frustration (for example, when his managing partner asked him to do things outside his area of expertise). During the workday he tuned out of these feelings, causing them to spill over when he got home, tired and hungry, in the evening. By this time, a full day of overriding his body's feelings had escalated and was misdirected at his partner who was an easy target.

The ability to listen to your body cues and interpret what they are telling you is vital for knowing how you feel in any given moment in terms of your emotions and physical requirements. Without this, your self-awareness is low and you cannot know what steps to take to meet your needs.

Cues for the basic maintenance of your body include the urge to go to the bathroom, hunger (when you need to eat), or heavy limbs (when you need to rest). In burnout, there is often a disconnect that has stopped you tending to your needs. The technical word for poor interoception (the ability to feel and listen to sensations in the body) is alexithymia, and it is something that about one in ten people suffers with. There are a few possible reasons for this:

- **Neurodivergence:** There is research showing that people who are autistic or meet the criteria for ADHD (attention deficit hyperactivity disorder) may have difficulties with interoception.
- **Trauma:** If you've suffered from a lot of intense experiences, you may have become adept at avoiding your body signals without realizing.
- **Bowing to Outside Pressure:** External stresses and a general pattern in our culture of paying more attention to output and external features (such as how you look or whether you completed a task on time), rather than listening to what you need, have trained you to stop tuning in to those messages. For example, if you consistently override the physical sensations of being hungry in order to finish your work, you might eventually stop being attuned to your body's signals.

When you fail to respond to the basic cues of your body, your emotions will let you know about it. You might get agitated because you haven't been to the bathroom or taken a break. This is your body turning the volume up on its messages to get you to listen! An emotion can also be triggered by a situation that is outside your body, like being let down by a friend or over-whelmed by busyness. Your emotions might be telling you that you need a quiet space to reflect or a reduction in stimulation, but you cannot know this if you are unaware of what emotions feel like in the body.

KNOWING WHAT TO LISTEN FOR

If you have not been tuned in to your body for a while, it can be helpful to see what you need to look out for. Each emotion has a physiological pattern in the body and an associated action urge. There is also a list of words to describe the intensity of the emotion. While noticing the emotion in your body is helpful, giving it a name can also improve self-awareness and make it slightly easier to see what you need.

Emotion	Words	Feeling in Body	Action Urge
Fear	Worried Anxious Overwhelmed	Tension Butterflies in stomach Nauseous Trembling or shivering Dry mouth Heart racing Shortness of breath Hot or flushed	Rush to safety or to fix an unresolved issue
Sadness	Empty Lonely Depressed	Heaviness Sinking or heavy feeling in chest Drooping muscles (e.g., shoulders)	Withdraw to "lick your wounds" or get support Seek out a way to restore what's been lost
Shame	Rejected Humiliated Inferior	Hot Tense Sunken or droopy muscles	Withdraw Hide Be submissive

Emotion	Words	Feeling in Body	Action Urge
Anger	Irritated Frustrated Violated	Hot Tension—in chest and especially facial muscles Shaking	Redress an injustice
Joy	Peaceful Excited Confident	Light Warm Energized or peacefully still	Connect with others

How to Start Listening to Your Body Again

- **Mindfulness:** This is one of the best ways to strengthen this listening muscle. The box on page 183 gives you a starter kit for this practice.
- **Yoga:** This gives you the benefits of mindfulness in addition to breath work and gentle movement of your body that help shift you through your sympathetic nervous system back to your green mode. You are actively guided to listen to your body. By moving in synchrony with the breath and focusing on any sensations you feel, you can build a connection with your body and improve interoception.
- **Check-Ins:** When there is a big breakdown in interoception, manually setting up check-ins throughout the day by using alarms on your phone can be a good reminder. Try to time these alarms during the transition parts of your day—for example, on clinic mornings I do a check-in between my therapy sessions. Once you hear the reminder, do this: Mentally scan your body from your head through your face, neck, shoulders, torso, abdomen, and down into your legs and feet. Ask yourself what you notice both inside and out. When I do this as I'm working, I often realize how deeply I'm frowning or how hunched my shoulders have become, and I can then stretch out to relieve some stress. But also be aware that it is perfectly acceptable to notice that there is nothing to notice! When we are calm and content, the body sensations are often more of a whisper, but it is still helpful to be

aware of the absence or quieter sensations so you can recognize moments of calm and glimmers to lean into. To enhance these short check-ins, I'd recommend practicing some longer mindful body scans. The guided meditations on YouTube by Dr. Mark Williams are a good option for this (see the Resources section on page 267).

- **Heart-Rate Experiment:** If you want to deliberately train yourself to notice your sympathetic nervous system (amber) response, this is an interesting exercise to try out. Use a biofeedback app (see pages 99–100 for examples) to measure your resting heart rate, or count the beats manually on a pulse point, then—safely, within the limits of your physical health—do something for a minute that elevates your heart rate, like jogging up and down the stairs or jumping jacks. Check your heart rate again and ask yourself what else you can feel in your body. Exercise like this can mimic the body's elevated stress reaction. Now practice some exercises from Chapter 5, like breathing, tapping, or visualizing. Notice what impact this has on your body and heart rate. This will help you to become attuned to your attempts to support your stress and gain an awareness of what green mode feels like.

What to Do Once You've Tuned In to Your
Body and Associated Feelings
Many people judge themselves harshly when they experience negative emotions like annoyance or when they feel upset, which adds another layer to the stress. Tuning in compassionately to your emotions involves recognizing that they play an important role in communicating your needs in any given situation. It is part of the human experience to feel these things, and all feelings should be given space and listened to. Anger is an emotion that can be particularly out of tune in burnout, so this gets special attention in the box on page 178.

Journaling can be a good way of figuring out which emotion is present and what purpose it has. Why not buy yourself a new "private" notebook to do this? Here are some prompts to get you started:

- Which emotion(s) am I feeling right now?
- What am I noticing in my body to show me that these emotions are here?
- Am I trying to avoid any of these emotions?
- If yes, why?
- What is this emotion saying that I need or need to do?

What If You Don't Like What You're Feeling?
This is the exact reason why you often lose touch with your emotions—because they are so unpleasant to sit with and are accompanied by your inner critic: thoughts where you put yourself down or you tell yourself you've failed or that you aren't entitled to feel these things. What we are trying to avoid here is reliance on the unhealthy protective strategies that push you further into burnout (people-pleasing, perfectionism, and getting busy again), and Chapter 11 will equip you with the compassionate alternatives.

TUNING IN TO ANGER

Anika told me she didn't ever feel angry. She never really had. At both home and work she was the one everyone relied on and went to; she was always warm and helpful and would put aside what she was doing to be available. We explored other words for anger to see what resonated—like irritation, frustration, and annoyance—but, again, she told me she rarely felt these things. However, what did resonate with her were the behaviors often associated with anger, such as being impatient (usually with herself), ruminating on problems, and criticizing herself.

Exploring the times when she got impatient with herself, she gave an example of needing to rush a staff change because she had helped someone with a last-minute request. Anika struggled with boundaries (such as letting this person know she could only offer five minutes rather than twenty) because she was unable to tune in to her anger. Her impatience was, in fact, her body telling her that someone had overstepped the mark by making excessive demands on her time and emotional energy (something they were clueless about because Anika gave off so many cues of friendliness). She was so adept at pushing anger away that she wasn't paying attention to what it was trying to tell her about her own needs. But overriding anger only worked up to a point because it was coming out in other subtler ways.

What Kinds of Problems Might We Get with Anger?
Anger is often pushed down because it is not considered an acceptable emotion to feel or show. Typical reasons for this might be a child having witnessed strong expressions of anger by adults that were scary and/or undercontrolled. They may then fear that this is inside them, too, and that it could cause damage if they let it bubble up to the surface. Similarly, if you were punished for expressing anger as a child you may have become accustomed to overriding this feeling. From a child's perspective it's safer to do this and maintain their attachment relationship with their primary caregiver than to risk being cast out of the family. For these people anger might feel genuinely absent.

Absence of anger, or an inability to tune in to it, may be very relevant in burnout. Without anger reminding you when the external pressures you face have become too much or unjust, you will continue to attempt to operate

179

without addressing them. Of course, you also may have had the damaging experience of feeling angry and being blocked from your attempts to act on this which can lead to learned helplessness. For example, if there isn't a safe way you can share the problems that make you unhappy at work or at home, you might give up trying. There have been many stories in the media of blocked unions and/or employees who don't feel psychologically safe (able to share problems) at work, so this is a common issue.

Without the wisdom of anger guiding you to uphold your limits, you end up without any boundaries or with very weak ones, caving in to requests at the drop of a hat. In Chapter 13 we will look at the assertiveness skills you might be missing to nurture your boundaries.

Another potential problem in burnout is when anger is *felt* but is overcontrolled, meaning there is no overt expression to others, and instead you quietly seethe or ruminate for hours. This keeps your sympathetic (amber) mode revved up for longer and grinds you down.

Isn't Anger Dangerous?

Feeling anger is different than communicating it in an uncontrolled way. Yes, it can be intense, but there are ways of working through it without dangerous physical expression to yourself or others, such as the following:

- **A Good Cry:** If you are able to, crying releases the build-up of tension.
- **The Tools in Chapter 5:** These practices are great for discharging from amber mode.
- **Shouting into a Pillow or into the Wind:** If you live somewhere where shouting won't be alarming to others, it can be a good release.

- **Journal the Anger:** Writing down your feelings helps you release anger and also helps you better understand it. Open a notebook and just write. Don't overthink what you're writing; this is just for yourself. Ask yourself what was happening when you started to feel like this. What was your anger trying to tell you? What would you have liked to be different?

These methods are important because, while anger is a vital consultant to us and plays a role in alerting us to problems, it is not always the most skillful of negotiators. Anger fires us up with the motivation and energy to defend and fight (threat system) but it is not always able to produce the most effective outcome for a given situation. When you listen to the anger, move through the intense part of it by asking yourself what it's trying to tell you about your needs, then safely express it using the outlined ideas; then when the heat of it has died down, you can plan a more measured, and more often effective, response.

Signs That You Are Feeling Angry Underneath It All

If you feel that anger is often missing in your life, consider the following to see if anger might be lurking below the surface:

- You are sarcastic or cynical (a more bitter version of sarcasm), covering your annoyance with wit.
- You are passive-aggressive; you express your annoyance indirectly.
- You are self-critical, turning anger inward; you tell yourself that things are your fault or that you should have done better.

- You dwell on things that were unfair or where you were wronged; you can't let go of thinking or complaining about them to someone unrelated to the actual issue.

What If You Have Too Much Anger?

Sometimes you might get an outburst of rage when you are not expecting it and then be very hard on yourself. This is a sign of chronic unmet needs. Your anger has been overridden for so long that it has bubbled up like a pressure cooker suddenly in a moment of stress.

If you get a lot of these outbursts or regularly feel a simmering of anger, then it might be helpful to know that this emotion is so empowering that it can sometimes be used (inadvertently) as a defense when you feel vulnerable. For example, if you feel sad or lonely, this might be quickly swept under the carpet by anger coming to your defense. If you want to understand what is underneath your anger, you could try to journal it, focusing on these questions:

- Where do you feel anger in your body?
- What does this anger want you to know?
- What does the anger fear would happen if it wasn't fired up right now?
- What does anger want for you?
- Are there any memories linked to this angry part?

If you want to read more about anger, see the Resources section on page 267.

MINDFULNESS

Mindfulness is the practice of deliberately paying attention to the present moment without judgment, noticing what pulls your attention away from it and guiding it back to where you intended it to be. Over time, this practice does for attention and interoception what weightlifting does for muscles; it improves its strength so it can support you in your daily life and, in particular, when life gets heavy.

Here is the essence of how mindfulness works. We typically choose something in the present moment to anchor our attention, such as sensations in the body or the breath. When we do this, the following pattern arises*:

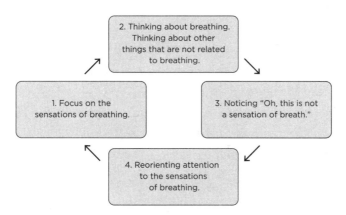

We are not aiming to clear the mind during mindfulness but to be aware of what has grabbed its attention—be that a thought, a noise, or a sensation in the body. The mind naturally wanders and continues to do so when you are doing a mindful practice. Noticing that it has wandered

*Adapted from #*What is Mindfulness?* by Dr. Tamara Russell, 2017, reprinted with permission.

and nonjudgmentally guiding it back to the anchor is the act of being mindful. We repeat this pattern many times during a mindfulness practice. This helps you to become aware of the sensations in your body, the patterns in your thoughts, and the ways in which your attention is often captured.

A Helpful Metaphor for Mindfulness: Leaves on a Stream

One of my favorite mindfulness practices is an image and also a handy metaphor. I often use this one to introduce people to mindfulness:

Close your eyes and allow yourself to find your soothing breathing rhythm. Take five to ten breaths like this to help your body slow down. Now bring to mind an image of a flowing river; this can be a place already known to you or one you're conjuring up in your mind for the purpose of this exercise. It is a quiet place where you can sit on the riverbank, watching the water float by.

On the surface of the water are leaves floating downstream. Your aim is to stay on this section of the riverbank, watching the water and leaves float past you. Every time you get a thought, image, worry, or memory, just imagine placing it on a leaf and watching it float past.

Repeat this over and over, placing anything that comes up in your mind on a leaf and letting it go. You may find you have recurring thoughts or thoughts about the practice itself (for example, "Am I doing this right?" or "I'm not getting any thoughts")—these are thoughts and can be put on leaves, too.

At times, you will realize that your attention has wandered off from the edge of the riverbank. In noticing this you have been mindful. Congratulate yourself and guide your attention back to the riverbank where you can be open to the next thought that comes into view. Continue in this way for three to five minutes.

This is just one of many mindful practices. Some people gel well with imagery, but others may not, so I have included a mindfulness of breath, too. Either way, I find that I can use this metaphor when I'm overthinking something by reminding myself that I can put it on a leaf rather than continuing to chew it over.

Mindfulness of Breath

Find somewhere comfortable to sit or lie for three to five minutes. If you are doing this unguided, I recommend setting a timer so that you aren't distracted by how long you have left. Allow your eyes to close, or rest them with a soft focus on a spot ahead of you. This reduces distractions. Now turn your attention to the sensations associated with breathing.

Notice the breath as it enters the body—the sensations at the nose or mouth. Notice how it is cooler on the way in and warmer on the way out.

Notice the sensations associated with breathing at the back of the throat and further down in the chest and abdomen— the small movements in the muscles and tendons—as the air enters and leaves your lungs. These sensations of your breath are your anchor in this moment. Every time your mind wanders off, gently guide it back to this. Focus on the words "this breath now" as you do so.

Continue for three to five minutes.

Troubleshooting

- **Mindfulness Is Making Me Feel Worse:** When you have spent a lot of time in amber mode, any mindfulness practice that involves being still goes against the fight-or-flight urgency in your body. What's more, you are being invited to direct attention *toward* experiences inside the body, like the breath or other sensations that you might be more accustomed to ignoring. If this is the case, you can try to engage with mindfulness of movement: focusing on sensations linked to movement like walking or yoga.

- **I Can't Clear My Mind:** This is a common misunderstanding in mindfulness, but the aim isn't actually to clear your mind. Rather, the aim is to be aware of what is passing through your mind and guiding it back to an anchor in the present moment. If you notice that you are getting a lot of thoughts, then you are being mindful of your thoughts, which is what we are aiming for! Now guide your attention with gentleness back to your anchor and you are doing mindfulness.

- **How This Can Help You Feel Better from Burnout:** The ability to notice where your attention is is the first step in choosing to interact with any given moment in a different way. It also supports you to be attuned to your body so you can be aware of the nervous-system gear that is currently in play.

- **I Find It Hard to Practice This:** Guided mindfulness is recommended for beginners. You can access mindful meditations for this via apps, but activities that have a mindful component can be a less formal way of getting started. For example, you can do any everyday activity mindfully, such as getting dressed, walking, or showering. Tune in to the sensations of the activity and when your mind wanders, gently guide it back to the sensations. This is called informal mindfulness. See page 270 for mindfulness resources.

Taking Your Mindfulness to the Next Level

There is a lot of research that shows that mindfulness can be helpful for anxiety and burnout. It can be taught as a stand-alone practice; the mindfulness-based stress reduction (MBSR) framework demonstrates consistently good evidence for its effectiveness. Mindfulness is also incorporated into other therapy approaches like CFT and acceptance and commitment therapy (ACT), both of which are good options for burnout.

Even with apps, those who are new to mindfulness can find it difficult to get into it without the support of a teacher or community. And there's also a possibility that those who are depressed can get stuck in ruminative thoughts. It's a tricky concept to come to terms with and hard to get a regular practice going without accountability. If you have tried mindfulness through an app and recognize that you would benefit from more guidance, then I highly recommend finding an MBSR group either online or locally.

Learning to tune in to your emotions and body sensations takes time. You may have spent many years overriding them, not want to listen for fear of what you may find, or feel like you cannot cope with any negativity. With practice, confidence in learning any new skill grows. This is true of your ability to notice sensations, to sit with any discomfort, and to understand what this is about. Over time, a better relationship with your body has the capacity to improve your burnout; you will be able to make more informed decisions about your needs and to slow down your responses rather than reacting from a place of avoidance. These are compassionate responses.

Chapter 11

TOOLS TO MANAGE YOUR INNER CRITIC

Just before her elastic band snapped and she was out sick with burnout, Anika's inner critic was running the show. It told her she would fail her staff if she didn't stay late to help; but then when she rushed home from work exhausted, it would berate her for missing dinner with the family. She couldn't win! It took her to task multiple times throughout the day: *I'm such an idiot. Why don't I leave work earlier? I'm a terrible mom! They must hate me.* Not only was she physically tired and emotionally spent from her nursing toils, but her inner critic layered on extra internal pressures that led to people-pleasing behaviors at the expense of self-care in her attempt to keep it at bay.

Anika started to use her mindfulness skills to notice the pattern of stress → rush about → self-attack. She began engaging the soothing tools from Chapter 5 and practicing mindfulness to break this cycle by allowing her nervous system to regulate. For example, she parked in the farthest garage at work so that she could do a brisk walk to her car after her nursing shift, allowing her to discharge the excess energy rather than letting it build up on the commute home. She also used her arrival home to sit for a few moments in the car and to give herself a hug, wrapping her arms tightly around her shoulders, reminding herself she was home and that she had done her best for the day and could let go of work now.

When we turn on ourselves in times of stress, as illustrated in Anika's case, we stimulate our already active threat system. It's like being hit by friendly fire when we are already under attack from the enemy (external pressures).

At such times, self-compassionate encouragement is an important way of relating to ourselves that counters the inner-critic voice. It has been shown to improve our heart-rate variability, giving us better stress management overall. When we do this, we are responding sensitively to our distress and this can slow down the urge to rush and strive with perfectionist, people-pleasing, and avoidance behaviors.

Compassionate encouragement involves softening the tone of your inner dialogue (to activate your social-engagement system) and reminding yourself of the ways in which the situation is genuinely hard rather than minimizing the stress you're under. For Anika, in this example, it meant reminding herself that she had an intense job and multiple roles (mom, nurse, and manager) and that it was important to her to do all of them well.

Think of times in the past when you had a compassionate, encouraging teacher compared to the one who just told you what you were getting wrong and became impatient. Which of those helped you persist and find enjoyment in the activity?

This chapter provides two exercises to respond to your inner critic in moments of stress and anxiety and two to strengthen your self-compassion muscle so that it's in fine shape when you need to draw on it.

RESPONDING TO YOUR INNER CRITIC IN THE MOMENT

Responding with compassion to your inner critic takes the heat out of the attack.

Imagery

Our bodies respond to both real-life and imaginary stimulation in the same way. For example, if I imagine one of my favorite meals in front of me—crispy roast potatoes fresh out of the oven with gravy oozing over them—this inviting thought causes my mouth to salivate and my stomach to rumble.

Something similar happens if we imagine a caring person showing us warmth and kindness. The social-engagement circuitry of the ventral vagal system is stimulated and oxytocin is released. Imagery like this is therefore a great tool for supporting your soothing system.

In Chapter 5, we introduced tapping in addition to calm-place imagery. You can build on this now with imagery linked to your social-engagement system. Try this next:

NURTURING-FIGURE VISUALIZATION

Before starting this exercise, take a moment to think of someone who has nurturing qualities. Either you have been on the receiving end of this yourself or you have seen them being nurturing toward others. You can go back in time and think of people who were previously in your life, even if it was only briefly, such as a teacher, aunt or uncle, friend, grandparent, or colleague. It can also be a figure from fiction, an animal, or a pet if you prefer.

Find somewhere calming to sit or lie and allow your breathing to find its soothing rhythm. Allow your muscles to relax; you may find it useful to tense them first and then relax them to help with this. Then soften your expression into that of someone who is showing warmth and kindness to someone who is upset.

Bring to mind the figure you identified earlier with nurturing qualities and think about these now. Notice what that figure looks like in the image. What is their facial expression like? How is their body language? Where are you in relation to them? Does it feel good to imagine any contact, such as a hug or reassurance from a hand on your arm or shoulder? Do they say anything? If so, notice their tone of voice and any turn of phrase that feels comforting. Notice how your body feels to be in the presence of this figure. Pay close attention, as you may find the experience of comfort in the body is subtler than threat-system emotions like anxiety and anger.

If you aren't used to engaging the imagination muscle, this might feel clunky at first, but it will improve with practice. Helpfully, it doesn't need to be a perfect image to start engaging the calming part of your nervous system; just the fact that you are sitting and attempting this exercise will be doing the same. Every time you practice, the new neural pathway you're trying to forge will be reinforced, so continue to do so and this will strengthen and become easier.

WHEN TO USE THIS TOOL

Nurturing imagery is a lovely, soothing option when we feel frustrated, upset, or down about something that has happened and are being hard on ourselves. It can be used as a stand-alone exercise or added in to strengthen the compassionate reasoning, too.

Here is how I use this for myself when I'm at work: Sometimes, I'll have a clinic that is particularly heavy going—one of those mornings when everyone I'm seeing for therapy seems to be having a particularly tough time. My motivation as a psychologist is to try to help others feel better, so, when everyone is stuck or in crisis at the same time, this sets off my threat response with self-attacking thoughts along the lines of: "I'm not cut out for this"; "they'd be better off with a different therapist"; or "if only I had done that extra training then I'd have better answers." When I use my compassionate imagery, I bring my mentor to mind—her warm and caring expressions and supportive words reminding me that therapy is hard and that I'm doing my best. I often add in a self-hug as I do this or slowly tap using the butterfly hug (see page 105).

RESPONDING TO NEGATIVE THOUGHTS

I've mentioned the inner critic a few times; this is a form of negative thinking. Negative thoughts have a direct impact on our emotions. For example, thinking, *I haven't revised enough to pass my exam* will make us feel upset and anxious, whereas *I nailed that presentation* will make us feel confident and happy. Negative thoughts are most likely to occur when we are in a difficult or stressful situation. It is the way our brains try to help us out (thanks, brain!) by warning us of all the dangers. The following table is a model from *The Compassionate Mind Workbook* by Elaine Beaumont and Chris Irons,* showing how our thinking shifts when we are in different modes:

	Threat-Based Thinking in Amber and Red Modes	Compassionate Thinking in Green Mode
Focus	Narrowly tied to the cause or trigger of the threat In anxiety, this is based on the things that could go wrong or possible dangers. In anger, this is based on things that are unfair or unjust. In shame, this is based on our own perceived failings.	Open and broad We are able to see the "wood for the trees."

---

*Reprinted with permission of the authors.

Form	Repetitive, ruminative, and lacking flexibility	Flexible and balanced We can notice but not overidentify with the thought.
Content	Nonrational, negative—"better safe than sorry"—overassessing risk and probability of harm	Underpinned by care, support, warmth, and compassion—balanced
Intent	Guided by nature of threat and specific threat emotion. For example: Intent to punish or seek revenge if based on anger Intent to avoid or appease if based on anxiety	Validation, empathy, and support Intention to be sensitive and helpful

Suraj, the architect, would go down a rabbit hole whenever he received a request for a design revision. He would get stuck in a low mood all day and would overcompensate by dropping his other projects to give the new version his full attention. He worried that the customer wished they'd been given a more experienced architect who could get it right the first time and that his manager thought he was bad at his job. These thoughts could spiral to even more unhelpful imagined places, such as getting fired and being unable to find another job.

Do you recognize how liberated you feel from these types of thoughts when someone gives you a fresh perspective on them? While psychologists are always advocates for reaching out for emotional support, we also know how hard this is if you're unaccustomed to it or not in a supportive environment, in which case a good starting place is to learn how to compassionately respond to negative thoughts yourself. The idea is to approach thoughts as simply that—as thoughts rather than facts. They may or may not be facts, and, as you can see from the previous table, when you are in the threat system thoughts are more likely to be exaggerated in terms of perceived level of risk and how firmly you believe that bad things will happen.

Here are eight steps to help you respond with compassion to negative thoughts. You might find a journal or notepad useful for working through these.

- Once you have noticed that your emotions have shifted into amber or red mode, **ask yourself what was going on in the run-up to this**. Often, especially with the long-term stress we get in burnout, there is a whole plethora of stresses and it's helpful to remember just how much is going on for you. But see if you can get specific, too. Was there a particular situation that has made you feel like giving up or suddenly irritable? What was going on? Was anything said? By whom?

  In Suraj's example he might recognize that he was already working on many projects and was already stressed when the email arrived advising that revisions were required. The tone of the email was abrupt and the customer hadn't thought to share the parts of the drawings that they had liked either.

- Now it helps to try to **identify what the threat-focused thoughts are** that you need to respond to. Ask or journal these questions: What went through my mind? What concerns do I have about how others are thinking of me? What worries do I have about myself?

  Suraj's thoughts were focused on how the customer and manager perceived him and his fears about his future as an architect.

- **What emotion has followed** these thoughts? For example, anger, sadness, guilt, or anxiety. There is often a mix of emotions, and it can be helpful to identify them if you can.

Suraj felt annoyed (angry) with the customer for being unclear in the original brief. He also felt sad that his work hadn't been shown any appreciation, and there was high anxiety as a result of the worries about his career. He felt some sadness for being alone with the weight of all of this.

• This next step is important (so don't bypass it) because it activates the green mode of your nervous system: your soothing. You are going to **set the intention to be compassionate with yourself** before you try to consider alternative perspectives to this thought. Soften your facial and body muscles to take on a compassionate body language, take five to ten breaths with your soothing breathing rhythm, and, if you wish to, you can add in some gentle tapping or a visualization for a few moments, too. Bringing warmth and kindness to the foreground also helps your frontal lobes come back into play and gives you access to more flexible thinking.

With Suraj, we discussed how to do this at work. He practiced taking a few minutes away from his desk by the coffee maker in the kitchen. As the coffee brewed, he would use this time to tense and relax the muscles in his shoulders and arms (an abbreviation of the progressive muscle relaxation on page 107), then do ten slow breaths. He would then try to approach his desk with a softer facial expression, letting go of the frown that had built up moments before.

• **Validate your experience.** Imagine that you got caught in the rain on the way to meet a friend; a validating response from them would be, "That's annoying. You poor thing. You must be so uncomfortable to be wet." Notice how that feels compared with an invalidating response such as, "You don't look too wet to me." We often invalidate our upset feelings, minimizing the impact they've had on us. A simple statement such as *It's understandable that I feel like this right now* is enough to connect to this.

Validating Suraj's experience in this example might involve acknowledging that his feeling of being upset is valid given how hard he has worked, how much he cares about providing good customer service, and how his efforts have not been appreciated.

- Next, you can **ask yourself balancing questions** that will stimulate and draw on your green mode. This isn't easy, and you might notice your threat-based brain resisting, but it gets a bit easier with practice and the steps before this will help pave the way, too:
  - How would I look at this situation if I didn't feel stressed and annoyed?

    Suraj: I'd remember that revisions are a very normal and expected part of the process. I don't live inside my customer's head, so it's impossible to capture everything they hope for in the first take.
  - What would I say to a friend with this issue?

    Suraj: I'd tell my friend that this is a tricky job and it's impossible to please everyone all the time. I'd remind them of the great projects they've done, too.
  - Am I applying the same rules to myself that I apply to others? For example, do I have perfectionist rules that I need to achieve a certain standard? Am I taking on more responsibility for others than I need to?

    Suraj: I don't expect others to sail through projects without revisions, so yes I'm probably setting myself unrealistic standards here.
  - Are there explanations that might account for the situation that I'm not thinking of?

Suraj: The customer may have been abrupt because they have a deadline. They also don't realize how much time goes into the work.

- **Bring to mind other times you've dealt with similar issues**. When you are in threat mode, you tend to underestimate your ability to cope or to come out the other side. You can use the imagery muscle to help you connect with your resilience and inner resources that help you to cope.

   Suraj brought to mind the big project he'd completed the previous month. Despite several back-and-forths with the customer, he had eventually delivered a design they'd been delighted with. Remembering this reminded him that he was capable and that setbacks were part of the process that he *could* get through.

- What would be **the compassionate thing to do next** given all of this? This is about moving the thought balancing into a practical space of being effective.

   Suraj felt that the compassionate way forward would be to let his manager know that he needed extra time for his other work given the new request. He also decided to share his frustration with a colleague who'd worked with this client before. His colleague was able to commiserate that the client tended to be quite pedantic on the run-up to deadlines, and it could feel hard to be on the receiving end of that. Suraj felt validated and his feelings of failure reduced.

Compassionate reasoning isn't easy. It takes practice. Our threat mode is so urgent and demanding, it will throw out more negative thoughts that try to convince us that it won't work or extra problems that start with *Yes, but...* The aim here is to use your compassionate attention to direct yourself toward what would be most helpful. Asking yourself, *How can I help myself right now? What do I need?* can help you stay oriented on this.

STRENGTHENING YOUR SELF-COMPASSION MUSCLE

Part of the reason why negative thoughts pipe up so frequently is that our brains naturally err toward "better safe than sorry" in a bid for safety. For example, if a friend texts you asking, "Can I call to talk for a minute?" your mind might generate (in the first instance) a worry that they have something bad to tell you. This is the nervous system's way of preparing for any defensive or avoidant actions that might be required to stay safe. Gratitude practices have been shown to be a good way of training ourselves to tune in to the good stuff and soften the hyper-focus of potential problems.

The Most Effective Gratitude Practice

Traditional gratitude exercises encourage listing positive things, like our life circumstances, events, and material possessions. While this is a sound starting place, it is only one form of gratitude practice, and research now offers us more insight into the most effective formats. In particular, there are differences between list-writing versus long-form letter-writing, the latter having longer-lasting impacts, and social versus nonsocial gratitude, which we will explore in more detail now.

The studies suggest that social gratitude (gratitude that we show to others or is shown from others toward us) is the more effective type because our social-engagement circuitry lights up (green mode), and we know from discussions in earlier chapters that this is powerful for regulating the nervous system. Essentially, when we tell someone that we feel grateful for something they've done for us, this strengthens the social bond.

But what does this actually look like in practice? A study where coworkers were asked to write letters of thanks to each other showed that being on the receiving end of these thoughtful words improved mood, with the participants' brain scans show-ing higher activation of the prefrontal cortex to back this up (brain areas associated with green mode). They concluded that a power-ful form of gratitude practice is to receive thanks from others.

While this gives us a lovely opportunity to help others feel better by expressing gratitude, it would not be an effective strat-egy to sit and wait for letters to be sent to us! Fortunately, a 2015 study led by Joel Wong showed that writing a letter of gratitude regularly can benefit the writer, too. Participants were assigned to one of three groups: Those in the first group were asked to write a gratitude letter to someone once a week; those in the second group were asked to write out their thoughts and feel-ings about a negative event (expressive writing); and those in the third group were the control group and had no writing task at all. Significant benefits in mental health lasting up to twelve weeks were found in those in the letter-writing group when compared with the other two. What's more, the benefits were retained even when the participants *didn't send* the letters to the addressees.

How to Build a Gratitude Practice into Your Life
- Once a week aim to think of someone who has supported you or done something you appreciated.
- Grab a notebook and address your writing to them ("Dear…").
- Write a page of thanks to them; don't worry about spelling because this is just for you (although you may choose to send it if you wish).
- Be specific about what they did or said that you found helpful.
- Write about the positive impact this has had on you.
- Try to focus on positive phrases; when Wong's researchers analyzed the letters, they found that those who used more posi-tive phrases experienced longer-lasting well-being.

What's important to note from the research is that the effects of gratitude practices on elevating mood and improving a sense of connection take time to build up (they might not be felt immediately) and are not long-lasting (they generally disappear if we stop them altogether). In much the same way that our bodies cannot store vitamin C and we need daily fruit and vegetables to get the benefits, it seems that we need to regularly practice gratitude to maintain optimum levels for our well-being, too.

WHAT TO DO IF YOU FEEL BLOCKED

This section is particularly relevant to you if you're feeling fatigue, heaviness, and "what's-the-point" thoughts to the extent that you're struggling to take even small steps to soothe yourself. This is a sign of where your nervous system is at right now, and you might need to go back to Chapter 5 and do some of the red-mode thawing-out exercises to bring a little more energy into your system (see page 96).

Remember the dogs in the learned-helplessness experiment (see the box on page 55)? They not only learned that they had no control, but their action of lying down indicated that they also had no *drive* to try to escape the electric shocks. To override the giving-up urges, the experimenters physically moved the dogs' legs to help them move to the "safe" part of the box. The dogs were being stimulated in an energizing way, and this helped to break the spell of learned helplessness.

What would be the equivalent for humans? You may have heard of the "power pose"—the idea that you can feel more confident before, say, an important, scary presentation by standing tall with your arms on your hips, head held high, and legs apart (like Wonder Woman). We can expose ourselves to uplifting stimulation through movements, empowering poses, sounds, smells, and tastes, and this can support the nervous system for a readiness for action. Research by compassionate mind experts has built on this by pairing energizing stimulation (via music) with compassionate-mind practices. The following steps are an adaptation of this that you can try if you are struggling with the drive to do the other exercises in this chapter. You will get the most benefit if you practice daily, but you might also want to precede other exercises with this one.

- Choose a song or a piece of music that you find uplifting and energizing.
- While playing the piece, slow down your breathing to find your soothing breathing rhythm.
- Imagine as you breathe in that you are breathing in a warm, compassionate light.
- As you breathe out, imagine the light you're sending into the world is also compassionate and joining up with the compassionate light of others in the world.

The other important point if you are stuck is that this might be a sign that you need more than self-help to get back on track. This is when a registered or licensed psychologist might be the next step.

If you feel you'd like to go deeper with some of the work in this chapter, see the Resources section on page 267, for more information.

Chapter 12

REBUILDING YOUR CONNECTIONS

Sarah was surrounded by people both at home and at work, all of whom had differing capacities for managing stress. During therapy she had become aware of how much she absorbed the distress of others and how the whole team suffered from the poor management skills of the current principal. She was planning to write a letter to the school administrators about it, but, while she plucked up the courage to do this, we considered some practical ways in which she could spread compassion and create a feeling of safety for herself and her stressed colleagues. She started a conversation in the group chat with the other teachers and suggested a fifteen-minute shared lunch on a Friday, telling everyone not to get perfectionist about what they planned to bring and that it was more than acceptable to show up with just a bag of chips to share—the aim being simply to help each other take breaks. And only conversations about non-work-related stuff would be allowed! This intervention felt manageable because it was concrete, within her zone of influence, and something she had to do anyway (i.e., eat!), so she didn't feel she was taking too much time out of her schedule to fit it in.

We do not exist in a vacuum. We are enveloped by family, teams, friends, and organizations.

In Chapter 4 we considered the three Cs of safety in our environments that lead to our nervous system reacting with either green, amber, or red mode. These were context, connection, and choice. You were invited to look for "glimmers" at that point: the little cues of safety that you might otherwise miss and, of course, to lean into them. In this chapter, we consider how to go one step further; we look at how to take deliberate steps to create an environment around you that feels safer with the potential benefit that this can ripple out to others who share it.

As a reminder: When an environment feels safe, we stop being trapped in survival mode and can move through our nervous-system gears more easily. This doesn't mean that we won't feel external stressors anymore but that we have more ways of coping by pausing and staying mindful of how this triggers our inner critic. When everyone feels safe, it's easier to provide compassionate support to one another and to accept and lean into this when it's available.

Compassionate support is powerful. Research consistently shows that it protects from burnout, even in situations where teams are faced with the most demanding of stressors, such as human suffering (as is the case for emergency departments or mental-health units). Compassionate support creates psychological safety: the ability to share when we feel unhappy, worried, or undervalued or to ask for the support and resources we require to flourish.

In this chapter, we focus on some practical ways to improve the three Cs of safety in relation to the communities and systems that you spend the most time in (like your family or work team). You will have different levels of power in the different systems you are in, so I'd recommend picking the ones you have the most ability to influence for now.

If you are recovering from burnout, then the last thing you need is to take on the responsibility of saving everyone and instigating big community projects, so the ideas here are simply invitations to nudge compassion outward whenever the opportunity arises. Of course, if you have any sway with the budget-holders at work, then a good, evidence-based way of realizing this would be through group mindfulness or compassionate-mind training for all levels of staff. But if this isn't possible, don't be discouraged; see what ripple-out effects can be achieved with the following ideas instead.

CONTEXT

We need to try to create contexts that optimize our well-being, give us permission to take breaks, and allow us to connect.

Space
- Consider how the space in question can be configured in a way that maximizes safety cues: How can natural light be optimized? Could more plants or natural materials be used in the space?
- Create dedicated areas for social interactions that feel welcoming (see pages 76–80, where I talk about hygge and so on) and are also separate from reminders of work and stressors. If you're in an office, this might mean banning work from entering the break room—perhaps a friendly sign or email to the team to suggest that this space is reserved for staff downtime and connections around non-work-related topics. If there's nothing you can practically do about the space you're in, then get away from work by inviting a colleague for a walk or coffee.
- Think about ways that social spaces invite non-work-related, side-by-side interactions. These can feel less intense than sitting

opposite one another. I often find when I put a 500-piece puzzle out on a coffee table, people naturally congregate and talk as they look for pieces. Putting up a "show-and-tell" board and inviting people to share postcards of their vacations, photos, or flyers of things they are doing outside work can help stimulate conversation like this, too. Can you do anything like this in the places you spend time in?

- Create a soothing corner or "station" for anyone in the team or family to use: a place where you can put calming tools for moments when people are in stress, like a music system, fidget toys, a glitter jar, a mat for stretches, or a comfortable couch; or a wall displaying letters of gratitude or support from clients or managers; or coping statements that you need to hear when you've had a stressful day.

Permission Not to Be Busy

You may have experienced being determined following a vacation that you are going to stick to taking your lunch breaks yet found this commitment had disappeared a week later. If there is a culture of overworking and wearing busyness as a badge of honor, it can be hard to challenge this.

Change is hard and takes time. Can you find just one person whom you can pair up with to hold each other accountable for taking breaks? You should each ask the other if they have had lunch yet and remind them that they have permission to pause if they haven't. If you are a parent, the same applies but might require a text reminder or taking turns holding one another's babies while the other one rests.

Start small: If you never take a lunch break at all, then start with a five-minute break. Do this consistently for a few weeks, then build up to ten minutes. You need a lunch break if you are a parent or caregiver, too, whether on weekdays or weekends. It is reasonable to tell your kids that you are out of bounds for a period; even if you feel like you're doing nothing, you are not. Parents of young children who feel that this is almost impossible to do might find *French Children Don't Throw Food* by Pamela Druckerman a helpful read for learning more about how well children can cope with waiting.

Suggest a weekly get-together with your team or family and ring-fence the time. Valuing this will take a lot of effort at the start but will get easier once it becomes established.

CONNECTION

Rebuilding social connections might feel like an uphill battle at first because negative-feedback loops can occur between people who are stuck in a stressed-out system. A feedback loop is like a familiar dance between two people: When person A steps to the left, person B responds by stepping to the right. The ball's then back in person A's court and their reaction will be in response to what person B did and so on. When we are faced with highly stressful environments, feedback loops between two reactive individuals can increase the toxicity and feeling of being trapped and alone.

For example, here is a feedback loop between Suraj and his colleague Jake: Jake felt stressed by an impending deadline, so he began rushing his work → Suraj noticed and became frustrated as this wasn't the standard he liked, so he redid Jake's section of a report ↔ Jake was upset and felt that his work was not being valued and so withdrew from Suraj → Jake and Suraj both felt more disconnected and their stress increased.

Systems can have dysfunctional patterns and this is particularly likely if they are under high external stress. Plus, once burnout is in the system, it can reinforce negative-feedback loops. For example, if a burned-out individual has lost their energy and is on autopilot, they may not be fully engaging in conversations and may miss things. Colleagues might misunderstand this as indifference or believe they don't want to be bothered and therefore withdraw from them. Loops like this can get stuck and cause a downward spiral for those burned-out and for others around them.

Get to Know Each Other Again

If you have kids and are in a relationship, then you and your partner are in a mini-system of two with management duties of a home and family to run together. Or you might be part of a sibling team within your wider family and perhaps together you have to navigate parents who are tricky or becoming dependent on you.

Think of each mini-system you are in as your "team," even if you wouldn't call it that. How then can you build your team up to function well together? Stressors can often push you away from your team members due to those negative-feedback loops or cause you to turn on each other rather than remembering that you all have the same underlying wish or purpose. The magic ratio of positive to negative interaction for healthy relationships is five to one. This means that for every moment you've snapped or criticized each other you need five positive interactions to protect the health of your relationship. This ratio can be difficult when you are stuck in feedback loops due to high external pressures—even when it's "just" everyday life stuff.

If your interactions don't currently match the healthy five-to-one ratio, then a "team-building" event might help to reconnect and bring joy back into the relationship. This could be a coffee or meal out or a long walk. I appreciate that this might mean you need to recruit help from others, such as getting a babysitter or taking some vacation days. The important thing to remember is that many connection and compassionate practices require time; they cannot be squeezed in as an extra, as this makes it all much more stressful.

Once you've carved this time out, try to limit discussing household chores. Instead, explore your individual or joint interests. Have a conversation about podcasts or TV shows you've watched lately, and ask questions about things you've each done and what you'd like to spend more time doing in the coming months. I see my husband every day and we rarely get past the "what's-for-dinner?" and "we-need-to-book-a-plumber" type of conversations. Even though we are physically together, it's not quality time that makes me feel close to him. It's closeness that makes us feel more warmth and empathy for each other when problems arise. It allows compassion to flow toward others in our system (in this case the kids) and makes it easier for us to accept help from each other when it's needed because we feel safe enough to do so—all of which is supportive and protects against burnout.

The same is true at work: Setting up specific times for work chat means you can get to know the people around you more fully. This increases feelings of support and reduces loneliness. It also means you'll be more attuned the next time one of you feels low or stressed.

A practical tool I sometimes recommend to support individuals within their teams is the "Manual of Me" (see the Resources section on page 267). This is a website with a set of reflective questions about your preferences and things you find stressful. If you and your colleagues or family members all fill one out and then share responses, it can reduce the guesswork around what each of you needs when certain situations arise.

Space for Reflections

Many workplaces and homes do not create space in busy calendars for reflection. Reflections allow space for us to make sense of the emotions or decisions of our workload. When made together they can also emphasize the teamwork aspect of any difficulties that have arisen. Without this there's no opportunity to feed back what works well and what doesn't or to problem-solve together or share ideas about how to improve. Carving out a regular time for this allows people in the system to feel secure that they will have an opportunity to share what they think and feel. It makes everyone feel seen, heard, and valued.

In terms of teams trying to work together, it is important to think about how you can do this. Perhaps starting and ending the day with a short "meeting" with a recognizable format. For example, a morning check-in could be as simple as sharing what you're working on, what others around you need to know (resources you need, when you'll be taking a break, etc.), and any concerns. And an evening check-in could involve what went well, what was tricky, and thoughts about how to overcome any hurdles. Small and regular check-ins mean that problems don't turn into big hurdles. Some places of work offer this already, such as a more formal meeting where the challenges and successes of care are explored together.

In a workplace setting you might benefit from having an external psychological consultant coming in to hold this space for you; this can increase safety and ensures the meeting goes ahead. At home, a gentle, regular check-in could happen at breakfast or on the school commute, or it could be a conversation at dinner or before bed. During any check-ins, try to practice active *listening*; this involves being fully present in the conversation and listening to understand, not just to plan your response.

Gratitude
In the previous chapter, I gave you the science of effective gratitude, explaining how social gratitude is particularly effective for protecting your emotional well-being. Individuals in systems where gratitude isn't expressed feel unappreciated, meaning that

work becomes unrewarding. A small way to help you feel better, improve connection, and make someone else feel good is to express gratitude to the people around you.

If this doesn't come naturally to you, it's a sign that you've missed out on this being shown to you in your life. But like all the skills in this book for managing your emotions, gratitude is a skill that can be learned at any age with practice.

GRATITUDE MYTHS
- You shouldn't thank people for things they should be doing anyway.
- You will spoil people and they'll get bigheaded.
- Gratitude needs to be a grand gesture.

GRATITUDE FACTS
- People will feel seen and their hard work appreciated if they're thanked for the things they do all the time; this improves job satisfaction.
- People don't get bigheaded from gratitude; in fact, many will minimize their contribution by saying things like, "Oh, it was nothing"—but this doesn't mean your attempt to express gratitude isn't worthwhile. They may not be able to soak it up in the moment, but they may come back to savor your comment when they are ready.
- Little-and-often gratitude is better than waiting for months and then doing a grand gesture.

HOW TO GET STARTED
- Think of someone who was part of your day today. This could be your kids, your partner, your kids' teacher, or a colleague at work.
- What everyday thing did they do that, if you pause to consider it, was a nice thing (possibly even a glimmer)? For example, did

your child come downstairs dressed and ready for breakfast? Did your partner make you a cup of coffee? Did your child's teacher smile and wait at the classroom door to welcome them?

- Pause (even just for a moment) and connect with the feeling that this person is in your life and what their gesture meant to you.
- Smile at them and try saying something that reflects your feelings, such as, "I love it when you come down dressed and ready for the day, thank you"; or "I don't always say it but I do appreciate when you bring me my morning cup of coffee"; or "I love how you help out [insert child's name] every morning—thank you for taking the time to stand by the door like this."
- Notice if they try to push the appreciation away, but know that this is not a reflection on you or what you've said.

CHOICE

Bearing in mind there is a sweet spot for choice—too many options feel overwhelming while too few make us feel trapped— try to find the small things you have choice over.

In acceptance and commitment therapy we explore a client's perception of their choices. Even when they feel like they have no options, trapped by a busy schedule or over- whelmed by racing thoughts, we look at the small choices they can make to work toward that sweet spot. For example, you can still choose to move your body in a certain way, such as stretching or slowing your breath or specifically directing your attention to something else, like shifting a worrisome thought onto a new activity. Perhaps you have choice over which project you start first or how work is delegated or even where you do your work.

If there is someone you can pair up with as your accountabil- ity buddy, you can each notice when the other reverts into old unhealthy habits that led to burn out. An accountability buddy can see and voice alternative options more easily for another person feeling overwhelmed or trapped.

If creating choices entails additional work or research, such as establishing who to delegate to or who to contact, an accountability buddy can see these routes more obviously than someone stuck behind the barrier of stress and anxiety.

To empower your choices in larger organizations where protocols can reduce choice, joining forces helps because many voices are more likely to be heard. When you are feeling exhausted from doing it on your own, syncing with others who want the same thing can soothe your nervous system.

Choosing How You Hold Others in Your Mind

When we are stressed we might have more negative thoughts about others. For example, we are more likely to attribute someone's upsetting behavior to an internal cause ("he's late because he is selfish") rather than an external cause ("he's late; maybe it was bad traffic"). It might be hard to imagine that we have choice over the way people are held in our mind, but we do.

There is a technique that can help our compassion flow toward others in our system which softens our thoughts toward them and encourages more acceptance and understanding. This technique is called Loving-Kindness meditation. Here is how to do it: Begin by directing the compassion toward yourself; slow your breathing down, place your hands on your heart, and say the words (or variations that suit you), "May I be happy, may I be safe, and may I be peaceful." Then turn the compassion toward others in your system: Bring them to mind, slow your breathing, and say to yourself the words, "May you be happy, may you be safe, and may you be peaceful." Start with someone you deeply care about (a person in your family or friend), then repeat with someone you feel more neutral about (like a bus driver or a colleague), then someone you are experiencing difficulty with at the moment (a person you've had a disagreement with). This practice may feel hard at first, but rehearsing it a few times a week will help you cultivate this flow of compassion.

We will look more closely at the personal choices you can turn toward in Part 4.

Part 4

POST-BURNOUT GROWTH

In trauma work, we talk about post-traumatic growth: the process of coming back stronger after adversity by embracing your relationships, appreciating new elements of life, and becoming open to making positive changes. Research suggests that about 50–70 percent of people experience this, with those who are open to reconsidering their belief systems being among the ones who are more likely to do so. We can apply the learnings from post-traumatic growth to burnout. I refer to this as post-burnout growth.

Chapter 13

SETTING THE GROUNDWORK

When Scott's creativity, energy, and enthusiasm dried up, it threw him. His business was his pride and joy, but feeling entrapped and ground down by it was not part of the original business plan! The heaviness he felt was familiar, though; he realized he'd felt like this in the run-up to his awful "nervous breakdown" (as his wife called it) during his old corporate job. That period had been intense. One morning after months of late nights and a sense of floating through the days in a haze, he had woken up, felt sluggish, and was unable to gulp down his morning coffee to get out early. And, more worryingly, he had been temporarily unable to speak. He'd taken a period of leave which had led to the big decision to hand in his notice and start his own project. He wanted the freedom to make decisions and manage his own time, so to recognize that the signs of burnout were now back again was startling. Maybe he needed to make more changes than just his employer? Maybe he needed to change up his relationship with work altogether?

Burnout can shift your fundamental view of yourself and the world. This is central to how you interact with others and how you apply yourself to activities and to your hopes and dreams for yourself. For your self-view or worldview to shift on its axis is a big deal.

Many people describe feeling disillusioned with their careers, managers, support networks, and organizations after burnout. Perhaps you recall being let down repeatedly or gaslit for months or even years, made to believe you were a failure rather than being offered the right resources to do the job effectively? This can affect your sense of trust in others, making it tricky to put in those healthy boundaries that everyone talks about. It takes gentle persistence to rebuild from this.

It can be quite a shock to learn that your body *cannot* keep going no matter what or that the "super mom" or "super dad" identity that defined you has collapsed. I once worked with someone who was known as (the equivalent of) Super Simon—the nickname his colleagues and family gave him because he put in such long hours and was so reliable. Part of why he took so long to recover from his burnout was because he felt that this fundamental part of his identity had become irretrievably lost. Without the Super bit, he was "just" Simon, and that made him feel like no one because his self-worth was so dependent on achievements. His therapy was about understanding who Simon was without relying on the Super part. And this was where he was able to discover aspects of himself that the Super part had obscured: his connection with nature, his love of podcast comedies, and his relationship with his wife. In doing so, he experienced positive personal growth beyond his old narrow identity.

RECONNECTING TO YOUR CORE VALUES

Shifts caused by burnout can offer an opportunity for post-burnout growth similar to Simon's. "Growth" in this regard means making changes that not only protect us from further burnout but enable us to live life more fully. But change is hard! We all have our old ways of doing things that feel familiar and easy because the years of repetition have deeply embedded the neural networks in long-term procedural memory. Establishing alternative behaviors involves going against the grain to lay down new neural networks until the new, healthier behaviors have become habits.

Doing hard things like this is made a little easier when we have a strong connection with our values—principles that govern how we act and give our life meaning.

Our daily activities are often dictated by our to-do lists, comprising of small goals we want to check off in the pursuit of bigger goals, such as completing a project, gaining a qualification, or getting a promotion. Goals like these are different than values. Values are ideas about how we want to live our life rather than a concrete outcome. Think of your values as the needle on a compass pointing toward the direction you want to be traveling. When your daily actions match your values, you tend to feel fulfilled and purposeful. Your values are the positive motivators of a healthy drive system, but they often get lost during the chronic stress of burnout when your overactive threat system has taken over.

How Can You Reconnect to Your Positive Motivators (Values)?
To make this more manageable, it's helpful to think in terms of the different domains of your life. In burnout, there has often been a strict focus on one domain (such as work or studying), where you have overapplied yourself and neglected other domains. Being reminded of all the richness available within the possible domains of your life is a very important starting point.

This approach to values is taken from ACT. Have a look at the domains outlined in the following table and take time to journal the associated questions to start assessing your values.* Well-being is all about balance, so notice any urges to skip a domain (unless it's not relevant, like parenting), and try to spend a little time on this.

Domain	Questions
Family	What sort of sibling, parent, son, or daughter would you like to be? Which qualities would you like to bring to these relationships?
Intimate Relationships	What sort of relationship do you want to build with your partner?
Friendships	If you could be the best friend possible, what would you be doing?
Parenting	What qualities would you like to have as you parent your child or children? How would you behave as the "ideal you"?
Career and Employment	What do you value about work and what would make it more meaningful? What sort of work relations would you like to build?
Education and Personal Development	What new skills or knowledge would you like to learn?
Recreation, Fun, and Leisure	What do you enjoy doing? How would you spend your time if no one was looking?
Spirituality (the meaning of this is flexible, such as cyclical living, being in nature, or following a more formal spiritual path)	What is important to you in this area?
Community Life	How do you want to contribute to your community? Which environments do you like to spend time in?
Health and Caring for Your Body	How do you want to look after yourself in terms of diet, sleep, and exercise?

*Adapted from a values worksheet by Russ Harris, available on https://thehappinesstrap.com/upimages/Values_Questionnaire.pdf, printed with permission.

As you explore these questions, you might find that you answer some of them with feelings: "I want to feel happy," or with goals: "I want to be good at my job." These aren't values you can live by. To uncover what those are from the answers you have given, you'll need to follow up by asking yourself: "If I was good at my job, how would I be acting?" In my job as a psychologist, I'd answer that question like this: "I'd be *present* and *compassionate* toward my clients. I'd be *connected* with other professionals and *creative* in my projects."

Here are some values that might help you with this exercise (it is not an exhaustive list):

Adventurous	Courageous	Friendly	Independence	Patient
Accepting	Creative	Fun	Intimacy	Present
Authentic	Curious	Flexible	Industrious	Respectful
Beauty	Dependable	Generosity	Justice	Self-Development
Caring	Equality	Gratitude	Kind	Self-Aware
Challenge	Empowerment	Honest	Loving	Spiritual
Compassionate	Forgiving	Humor	Mindful	Supportive
Connected	Faithful	Healthy	Open	Trustworthy
Contributing	Fitness			

All this information about your values is useful for post-burnout growth in three ways:

1. It can help you to get clear on the ways in which you're neglecting domains that could give you balance. For example, entrepreneur Scott was neglecting almost all the domains except work and personal development. He simply wasn't spending any time thinking about other areas, although his pangs of guilt were alerting him to the fact that he wasn't aligned with all his values.

2. It can remind you of the ways in which you want to show up in the areas of life where you *do* currently spend a lot of time.

For example, even though Scott spent a lot of time working, he often wasn't doing this in a way that aligned with *all* his values. He was *industrious*, yes, but he was not as *open* or *creative* as he wished to be. In fact, he was often the opposite of these because he was stressed and reactive. This didn't feel good. Taking the time to consider the questions in the career section combined with the following steps allowed Scott to think through the changes needed to make work more fulfilling— such as getting more support so he could free up time for creative thoughts again.

3. Values can be used as your foundation for making day-to-day decisions. If you feel that something is hard but will take you a step toward a value, then it is probably a good choice.

STEPS TOWARD VALUE-BASED LIVING

Ask yourself: Which domains from the table on page 220 are well connected to your values and which are not? Which of the neglected domains would help you get more balance into your life? Choose one to focus on.

Now you can take six steps toward creating meaningful goals related to this.

*Step 1: Write a Short Description of the Domain and
Value You've Identified and Want to Work On*
For example, *In the domain of friendship, I value being trustworthy, fun, and connected.*

*Step 2: Set Yourself a Mini-Goal That You
Can Carry Out Immediately*
What is the easiest small action you can do right now that would be a step toward this value? Where is the least friction in terms of practical things to arrange or worrisome thoughts

that arise? For example, you could send a voice note or text to a friend telling them that you're thinking of them or share something interesting that happened recently which reminded you of them.

Step 3: Plan Your Short-Term Goals
What small steps can you take this week that are consistent with this value? Goals are most successful when they are specific. For example, *tomorrow I'll text a few friends to see who is available for a catch-up during my Friday lunch break.*

Step 4: Set Longer-Term Goals
Start to think bigger now. What challenges could you set for yourself that would take you closer to your value? Perhaps, *I will arrange a regular meet-up with my friend for a walk.* Or, *I will invite my friend to come and stay for a weekend.*

Step 5: Life-Changing Goals
This might sound dramatic but if you've hit severe burnout, this step is important and may be sorely needed. It can be very hard to do this when you are still in the thick of burnout because your ability to imagine a different reality to right now is harder for a burned-out brain.

Imagine you are meeting yourself in five years' time, and in this future you have the life you'd love for yourself. What are they doing? Who are they surrounded by? What have they achieved? What do they have going for them in their life that you yearn for? Imagine they are free of the expectations or judgments of others: What has that freed up for them to go and do?

Journal these questions, talk to others, and take inspiration from books, movies, and podcasts. See where this leads. Allow yourself to be free and playful with it and to dream big. You may have a dream of starting a new business in an area that's completely new to you; you may dream of living in a new place or creating something awesome. Any of these can be the inspiration that helps guide your steps.

Step 6: Visualize How You Will Achieve This
Research shows that visualizing an outcome helps us to achieve it—for example, an athlete taking the time to imagine the course they are due to run and mentally rehearsing when they will bend into the curve of the track or shift their pace for obstacles.

Close your eyes and imagine taking the steps you need to move toward your bigger goal. When you encounter obstacles or worrisome thoughts, give yourself permission to consider how you'd deal with these. Say to yourself, *I can handle this*, then picture how you'd do so. Run this like a movie image through your head until you get to the end. You can repeat this if you wish.

This can be strengthened with bilateral tapping (see page 105).

Putting It into Action
Now you are ready to take concrete action, so consider which resources you'll need. These might include practical things, such as a new diary or habit-tracking app, or emotional resources, like an accountability buddy or a set of positive reminders (affirmations or your visualization). Put these where you have easy access to them. (See the Resources section on page 267 for ideas.)

Here is an example of what you are aiming for, showing the difference between values, goals, and actions.

Domain	Values	Goals	Actions
Career and Work	Creativity Industrious Dependable	To become a supervisor this year To do a supervising training for this	Research supervisor trainings Enroll
Health and Body	Fitness Fun Empowerment Independence	To start jogging regularly To enter my first 5K	Buy proper running shoes Download the "Couch to 5K" app Go for my first jog

Remember, you can check off a goal but you cannot check off a value. Taking small, daily actions aligned with your values will help you recover from burnout by building a meaningful life. If your identity was rocked by burnout, you can choose the values that support your identity in a fuller way. For example, Super Simon valued being *loving, adventurous*, and *fun*. In his burnout recovery, he could see how the value of being *industrious* had dominanted and how one regular action could help him live with his *adventurous* value at center stage, such as taking his dog to beaches and woodlands rather than the same old walk around the block.

What If You Have Two Values That Compete?
Anika valued being a *patient, loving*, and *present* mother, but she also wanted to be a *respectful, compassionate* manager who tended closely to her own *personal development*. Sometimes the two domains competed for her time, like when she was invited to attend a conference that would help keep her up to date for her management duties, but it was on a day off when she'd usually spend time with her kids. On the conference day she therefore tried to find a small action that allowed her to move toward her value of being a patient, loving mother, even if only for a short time. For example, she avoided

turning on her phone until after breakfast and ensured that the kids had 100 percent of her attention before she headed off for the day.

What Will You Need to Sacrifice to Pursue Your Core Values?
This question might feel challenging at first glance, but if you give it proper thought it can be very liberating.

If you have become burned out, you have already made a sacrifice in pursuit of work-based goals or putting others first; you have sacrificed your health and well-being. If you start to reclaim these, you will need to give something else up to do so because you cannot squeeze anything more into the day. For example, Super Simon realized he was giving up his do-it-all identity, Anika realized she would have to give up the speedy pursuit of her next level of promotion, Suraj realized he'd have to give up trying to please everyone, and so on. You might even need to consider giving up something practical that has taken you a long time to get established, like your business or career, to pivot into something else that is more aligned with your values.

Don't let the sunk costs of your time and energy (things you've already done, the costs of which cannot be recovered, such as training or qualifications) prevent you from giving this real thought. If you start over, you aren't starting from scratch; you're just starting from experience. And try to keep in mind the bigger picture: In five years' time, what would it mean for you if you don't make these changes? And what would it mean for you if you do? Journal these questions.

SELF-CARE REBRAND: VALUING *MYSELF*

Since you are reading this book and tending to your needs during or following an episode of burnout, I'm going to make an assumption that you have a core value around your health, self-care, or self-development. Sadly, the phrase "self-care" has an image problem; it is often thought of as a luxury that people in the real world have no time for, and there is also a misconception that it should instantly feel good. In fact, self-care is about basic body, brain, and life maintenance. It is the small, regular habits that help you create a life that you don't regularly want to escape from. The cumulative effect will be positive but you might not get a big hit of happy hormones from one-off self-care activities.

What if we take the work you've done on your values in this chapter and rebrand self-care as "valuing myself" instead? If you've neglected yourself for a while, it can be helpful to go back to basics with what this should regularly look like:

Daily

Getting up; tending to your personal hygiene; eating nutritious food; moving your body; connecting with others; resting (time when you're not creating, producing, doing, or sleeping); a practice for your emotional health (even if it's only short), like mindfulness, breathing, placing your hand on your heart, or getting enough sleep.

Weekly

Getting variety into your week in terms of what you're working on, what you eat, and how you move; making sure you have organized the resources you need to function well, like clean clothes, food in the fridge, or a decluttered space;

including reflective time, like planning or journaling, checking in with how you feel and are doing, plus thinking about what's coming up and what you might need.

Monthly

Attending any health appointments; making sure you have what you need, such as season-appropriate clothes, getting bills paid, etc.; taking a proper break from work (this might be from the kids or dependents) and making a date for the next one so you have it scheduled; having some sort of "team-building" time to properly connect with others outside of life and work duties; having some sort of project that fills you up, excites you, or makes you feel good—for example, a craft or do-it-yourself project, reading a book, training the dog to sit—anything that gives your brain a break and anchors it.

Some people find it helpful to schedule a time in the day when they will do these types of "valuing-me" activities. Put a fifteen-minute weekly slot in your calendar if that helps you. Essentially, this cannot be squeezed in as an extra; change won't happen unless you put this in and then schedule all your other activities around it.

Once you have a sense of your values, you can start to get into the practical ways in which you can thrive in post-burnout which we will cover in the final chapter.

Chapter 14

A TOOLKIT FOR THRIVING

Remember how hard Anika was on herself when she got home late from work each night and missed her kids' bedtime?

Self-compassion is more than simply talking kindly to ourselves and soothing our distress. It's also about *taking consistent actions* that will move us into a better place: post-burnout growth. In Anika's situation, this involved learning to listen to her body to work out what she needed and then learning what boundaries are and how to uphold them (which meant having some tricky conversations with colleagues) so she could protect her time and energy.

For Scott, post-burnout growth meant learning to slow down and make decisions from a measured place rather than his typical fast reactions.

Sarah learned how to wind down from work in the evenings so she could follow her other values, like yoga and friendships.

Suraj learned how to set more realistic standards for himself which made him feel less pressured.

The following practical ideas for post-burnout growth are the healthy-living tools you might be missing for setting boundaries and certain aspects of self-care. Some of them will feel challenging if they are new to you which is why you'll need some strong foundations in place to stick with them.

You might not need all the tools outlined here, but let's just take a look and then work out which you need to focus on.

LEARN YOUR PERSONAL SIGNS OF BURNOUT

Go back to Chapter 1 and review the Five Stages of Burnout on page 20 and the list of burnout symptoms on page 6. Identify the most recognizable two to three behaviors, thoughts, or physical reactions that you see in yourself. This will aid you to quickly identify signs that stress is building up and help you take prompt, positive action. If you feel able to, talk to your closest allies: your partner, family, or a close friend. Ask them if they've seen any signs that you are burned out that you may be less aware of and to highlight (compassionately) their concerns the next time they notice them.

LEARN HOW TO SLOW DOWN

Slowing down responses is particularly helpful when the demands facing you require your brain's higher-functioning capacities and measured decision-making. If there's no actual emergency, that urge to rush is actually a sign of a wrung-out nervous system. If you can hold this in mind, then you can use this sense of urgency as a sign that you need to pause. Slowing down, even if it's just through micro-pauses, allows the space to listen to your body and emotions, make careful decisions, and reconnect to your values before responding. Without this, you risk regretting your actions and perpetuating the boom-bust pattern that contributed to burnout in the first place.

How to Slow Down

Again, this is where mindfulness (see the box on page 183) plays a big role. Mindfulness allows you to step out of the content of the moment and take a bird's-eye view. Have you ever watched a "making-of"-style documentary or TV show where there is a voice-over describing what's happening and how decisions were made at certain points in the show's evolution? Regular mindful practice gives you this voice-over narrative. For example, one evening when I was making dinner after work, I was trying to remember a recipe while listening to the radio. My daughter was doing her homework at the kitchen table, every so often piping up with a math question, and then one of my other children came in to ask me where his Lego was and to moan about what I was cooking. Aargh…

Using my mindfulness, I was able to pause and notice how hot and stressed I was and that I was feeling a strong urge to snap at my unhappy child. Then the voice-over came on in my head and went something like this: *You are stressed, and you feel hot and tense; What would help you right now?* This small pause was enough to allow me to make two helpful decisions to remove some stimulation. First, I turned off the radio; second, I told my kids I needed to focus on one thing at a time, asserting a boundary. I told them I would answer their questions after I'd finished preparing dinner.

LEARN HOW TO SWITCH "OFF" FROM WORK

We often use the phrase "switching off" when we think about disengaging from work. However, the reality is that for many of us this is not a simple flick-of-the-switch process; a more helpful metaphor is to think of yourself as shifting down the gears as you might when driving.

Many people in burnout say they struggle with this, often believing that the "to-do" type thoughts their brain generates

231

during downtime are signaling that they should be acted on immediately. However, the truth is that your brain is a problem-solving machine, and if it's not currently engaged in a fixing task it will look for the next issue to fix. This means that your down-time can be filled with thoughts like, *I didn't email George back yet! I haven't bought a birthday present for Sasha yet! I need to pay the window cleaner!* And so on. Here are some techniques to help you with shifting down the gears:

- **Follow a Wind Down Routine:** Moving from working to non-working is a transition point of your day, so try to mark it as such. If you are leaving a place of work, perhaps you can start by tidying your work area so it's welcoming for the next day, stretching your arms, and closing down any computers or machines; line up some easy-listening podcasts, computer games, or books for your commute. If you are at home because you work remotely or are a caregiver, student, or parent, this is equally important. Decide what time you are "clocking off" from nonurgent duties, such as household chores, and if you get any thoughts of outstanding items, write them on your to-do list. Mark the end of your working day with a short walk, a shower, or by changing into some comfortable clothes. If you can, try to have a fifteen-minute period for yourself and imagine this to be your commute home when people often decompress. Listen to a podcast, call a friend, knit, read, or play a computer game or an instrument. Do anything that releases the pent-up stress hormones from being "on" and also signals to your body that you're coming to the end of your working day.
- **Remember That It Takes Time for New Routines Like This to Become Second Nature:** Expect it to take at least three to six weeks of effort before it gets easier.
- **Practice Mindfulness:** Yes, this again! When you've set an intention to wind down or do relaxing activities, mindfulness helps you

notice when you are being pulled into problem-focused thoughts and urges you to slip back into "doing mode."

- **Do Activities That Engage You:** Switching to a different engaging type of activity can tap into a fresh part of the brain and help your thinking brain let go of its to-do list. For example, creativity, playing games, sports, or hobbies.

- **Reduce Reminders of Work:** You get more doing-mode thoughts when your brain is reminded of work. This might be in the form of visual reminders (seeing a pile of laundry) or email notifications. If your work is separate from your home life, this might be easier, but you may also need to take some practical steps; for example, investing in a separate phone for work or asking your manager to fund this so you can switch it off and lock it away; taking work-related apps off your home screen; or signing out after hours if you cannot have a separate phone for work.

- **Home-Based Reminders:** I find hiding unfinished work helpful. I have a home office and shutting the door can be immensely useful. Otherwise I'm tempted to pop in as I'm walking past. When my kids were little and created a mess, I would push their toys into a pile and throw a blanket over it in the evening so I didn't need to look at the mess while watching TV. Having a comfy or quiet space that you reserve for relaxing can also be a lovely way of getting into the mental space for shifting down the gears.

LEARN WHAT REST REALLY MEANS

Burnout is the direct result of a lack of appropriate rest. Rest tends to get pigeonholed as the action of physically pausing and conserving energy levels. However, it is so much more than this. Imagine you are painting a rainbow and the colors are different pots of energy; violet might be physical energy, indigo might be emotional energy, and blue might be your brain or thinking energy. The joy of a rainbow is when all the colors shine brightly, and for this to happen you need to pace how much you dip into these pots of energy throughout the day and week.

How to Rest

The most helpful idea I've come across that has helped my own therapy clients is from psychologist Suzy Reading in her book *Rest to Reset* (see the Resources section on page 267). She offers a very practical model called the eight pillars of rest,* inviting you to consider the ways in which you have been spending your emotional and physical energy to work out what you might need in any given moment.

Resting doesn't need to be reserved for the end of the day. Take some time to think about the whole of your day and how you can make adjustments to get balance in the eight areas outlined here—even in small ways, such as walking during a meeting, stretching at transition points in your day, or calling a colleague to discuss an issue rather than emailing about it.

Movement ↔ **Stillness**

Have you moved much today? Do you need more movement if you've been sitting for long periods, or do you need stillness now?

Stimulation ↔ **A Break from Stimulation**

Have your senses been used a lot today? Which ones? If yes, how can you take a break from this; if no, what kind of stimulation will offer you balance?

High Energy Levels ↔ **A Soothing Dissipation of Energy**

Do you need something uplifting and energizing—a boost because you feel de-energized? Or are you carrying pent-up energy, feeling fidgety, and needing to allow this to dissipate?

---

*Reproduced with permission of Suzy Reading and Octopus Publishing through PLSclear.

Solitude ↔ **Being in the Company of Others**

Have you spent a while in solitude and could now benefit from the company of others; or have you spent the day socializing and need to be alone or with the comforting presence of a friend, partner, or pet?

Mindful Focus ↔ **A Free and Wandering Mind**

How has your brain been engaged? If you've been working mentally hard or absorbing content during a lecture or client calls, perhaps you need to give your mind space to decompress through something gentle or "easy," like listening to music or coloring.

Emotional Expression ↔ **A Break from Your Emotions**

Sometimes taking a break from emotional expression can be helpful; at other times you may have had to bottle them up in order to continue with other activities. Do you need to tune in and journal them now, or do you need to take a break from them?

Comfort and Ease ↔ **A Stretchy Challenge**

Has the day been humdrum and filled with monotony? Perhaps you need something fresh to sink your teeth into? Or perhaps you crave the familiarity of routine, your favorite spot on the couch, and a date with your book, phone, or TV?

Giving ↔ **Receiving**

Who has been on the receiving end of your attention? If you've been providing for others in your duties at work or at home, how can you yourself receive care now? Can you ask someone else to put the kids to bed or take up an offer of help when your initial urge is to decline? Or if you've spent all day disconnected from giving and would like to do this now, how can you give back—perhaps to your family or your local community?

LEARN HOW TO FALL ASLEEP

There's a common myth that sleep comes easily when you are exhausted. But in burnout you may have learned that this isn't the case. You are "tired but wired"—beyond exhaustion but unable to fall into a deep slumber. This is because the most important factor in falling asleep is actually feeling safe enough to do so. For our ancestors, this meant being safe from predators and other dangers; in modern times, this equates to nothing being required of you, aside from your nervous system needing to release enough of its stress hormones to shift down the gears into green mode. Chapter 5 provided practical exercises to practice regularly, but if you are focused specifically on getting sleep back on track, you'll need to combine those exercises with some viable steps:

- You need a wind down routine specific to bedtime. This doesn't need to be complicated or fancy. It might be simply watching some TV followed by putting on PJs and then reading a chapter of a book.
- A few years ago, the advice around technology and sleep was fairly black and white: Avoid all screens for a couple of hours before bed due to blue light emission which interrupts the production of the sleepy hormone, melatonin. Now, however, updated research suggests that not all screen time has the same negative impact on sleep onset, and, in fact, if the technology you're using helps you to relax—such as watching something on TV (i.e., passive consumption of media)—it might actually have a positive role. However, when your digital consumption is more active, like playing games, working, or commenting on social media posts, you'll more likely be in your amber mode which means you will need to allow time to wind back down from this usage. So: Factor in the type of screen time you're having, and if it's not the green

mode, relaxing type, make sure you stop early enough to switch into a more relaxing task before you turn off the light.

- The same advice goes for any activities that will stimulate your nervous system. If you want to journal, make sure you do this early enough in the evening so you aren't getting wound up.
- Keep a notebook by your bed in case your brain conjures up to-dos as you try to fall asleep. You can write them down to allow your brain to let go.
- Don't stay in bed if you cannot sleep after twenty minutes of trying; you will get stressed and then create a negative association with your bed. Get up and do something gentle and not stimulating. Then try to go back to bed again when you start to notice sleepiness.
- Use mindful practice and/or a progressive muscle relaxation once you're in bed. This sets the intention to fall asleep and tells your brain and body that you're ready to let go of stresses and worries.

LEARN WHAT BOUNDARIES LOOK LIKE AND HOW TO SET THEM

Boundaries are the invisible walls around your resources: your time, energy, beliefs, values, and body. You *should* have a sense of when a boundary has been crossed because your emotions pipe up to tell you in the form of anger (frustration or annoyance). But as I've already outlined (see the box on page 178), this is not always the case. The reality is that our culture prioritizes the boundaries of different people to varying degrees with a tendency toward caregiving roles being given less weight. This means that people who care for others are not always taught how to effectively put boundaries into place or given skills for reinstating them when they're violated.

When you don't consider which boundaries you need to stay balanced or take time to make them known to those around you, you not only risk being taken for granted and overworked but also have less of a buffer in place for life's challenges because you have spent all your energy or resources on others.

Moreover, if you fail to clearly communicate your boundaries, you can inadvertantly end up acting them out in ways that might be more passive-aggressive; for example, being sarcastic, avoiding responding, rushing a job, gossiping to others, or sighing and muttering to yourself when you are doing something you don't want to do.

How to Set Boundaries

The trick to setting boundaries is to get clarity on which you need and then to communicate them as clearly as possible to those who need to know. Many people are so unaccustomed to setting boundaries that they mistake assertiveness for aggression. However, if you politely state your wish, sticking to the facts unapologetically, this is clear and positive communication of a boundary. If you find this hard and worry about upsetting others, it can be helpful to think of a time when someone has clearly communicated a boundary to you and how it felt to be on the receiving end of this. Often there's a relief that you don't need to guess what the expectations are or that you're not going to mistakenly overstep the mark.

Which Boundaries Do You Need to Put in Place to Combat Your Burnout?

Psychotherapist and author of *Set Boundaries, Find Peace* Nedra Glover Tawwab explains that there are different areas of life in which you might require boundaries to improve your burnout, such as your finances (not paying for others' needs when you don't want to or don't have the means); emotions (not being responsible for others' emotions); time (clearly separating work and personal); and values (doing what you believe in, not what others want of you).

One of the biggest boundary violations in burnout is personal time. Many people have such shaky boundaries that they find it hard to separate when they are "on duty" for others from their personal time. Stronger boundaries can look like this:

- Keeping separate digital spaces for work and pleasure by using a different phone for work (if you can) and finding a place to lock it up for the night when you stop. Set an out-of-office email message to communicate this boundary to your colleagues and clients. Only use desktop versions of websites for work as much as you can (apps are all too easy to open on autopilot). If you need to use an app for work, schedule time for it in your diary—for example, "social media updates" or "online community management."

- Keeping separate spaces at home for work-related activities, like studying or working. If you don't have the luxury of space, this may involve being disciplined with tidying up after a work session which can be part of your wind down routine. Do you need to spend some time creating storage or decorating sections of a room to give part of it a work vibe and part of it a chill-out vibe?

- Setting an alarm for stopping work or having an accountability partner and arranging to call each other at a set point to ensure you've stopped.

- Having a regular routine with your breaks so everyone around you knows when you're enjoying your morning coffee, taking an after-dinner walk, or watching your favorite TV show alone.

Communicate Your New Boundaries with the People Around You
Start by setting a boundary with someone you have a good relationship with—someone who you know really respects you.

You might also benefit from telling them what you're doing and why. Explain that you're recovering from burnout and have realized how shaky some of your personal boundaries are so you're going to start communicating them more clearly from now on. The reason for starting this way is that you will encounter tricky feelings (anxiety and guilt are most common) and (probably) some pushback from people who aren't accustomed to you having boundaries in place. Responses can vary in how they look from more attacking "You always drove me in college. Why do I need to start taking the bus?" to apparent flattery "You're the right person for this job. You'll do it so well. I couldn't possibly imagine giving it to someone else."

Here is an overview of the steps you need to take to start setting boundaries with others:

- **Know What Your Needs and Values Are:** See Chapter 13 and also the first point in this chapter.
- **Clearly Communicate Boundaries to Others:** Talk directly to the person in question, keeping your body language open and nonthreatening and using eye contact and a steady voice that's neither too loud nor too quiet. Use "I" statements: "I need," "I would like it if…," etc. Keep the communication specific to one topic and without blame: "I know you'd like this done today but I have not allocated the time. I can do it tomorrow, though."
- **Ride Out the Tricky Emotions That Show Up:** While I've explained elsewhere in this book that you should be listening to the wisdom of your emotions, there are times when you might need to ride out emotions without allowing them to guide you. This is one of those situations. Anxiety and guilt will appear if you are doing something new and unfamiliar and also if you are going against the grain of what has been socially expected of you (even if you logically know that this isn't OK for your

well-being). Expect the anxiety and guilt and bring them along for the ride; these emotions will start to become less intense the more you become familiar with honoring your needs and values in addition to those of other people.

- **Stick to Your Guns When You Get Pushback:** People around you are going to lose the benefits they've received from your lack of boundaries. Your boss may need to recruit a new staff member if you stop working extra shifts; your partner may need to take on extra duties around the home or with childcare; your friends may need to start sharing the organizing of nights out rather than relying on you to do it all. As a result, you may notice some pushback from these people. Aggressive pushback is often easy to spot; this is when someone becomes verbally attacking or defensive. But in my experience, it's more common to get pushback that's more insidious and harder to stay strong in the face of. For example, ignoring your request which makes you feel awkward about stating it again; questioning your judgment ("Are you sure you can't make time?") which makes you doubt your boundary; emotionally blackmailing you with comments like, "It'll be annoying if you don't come" or "But you're so much better at doing this than I am; I'm going to mess it up." Notice this and label it as pushback.
- **Repeat:** Repeat steps 2–5 as necessary.
- **Remember to Praise and Thank People Who Accept Your New Boundaries:** Positive reinforcement will work wonders for maintaining this new way of relating and will make it easier for future boundary-setting, too.

How to Stick to Your Boundaries

Of course you can communicate boundaries but you will still be asked by others to do things, from staying late at work to driving someone home or helping a friend out. How do you manage to stick to your boundaries when requests like this come in?

THE TRAUMA OF BURNOUT

The most important element is to slow down your response. When you pause before responding you give yourself the time you need to check in with your emotions and needs. Practice offering a holding response along the lines of, "Can I think about this and let you know?"

Requests can trigger the insecure striver part of you. For example, people-pleasers will want to please the person with a quick response. If this is you, you will need to practice riding out any anxiety that arises (you can use tools from Chapter 5 if this gets intense).

I find professor and social worker Brené Brown's technique invaluable here. She wears a ring that she can spin around with her fingers. When someone asks her to do something, she pauses long enough to spin the ring three times while reminding herself to "Choose discomfort over resentment." By this she means that she will feel uncomfortable during the moment of pause or choosing to say no, but the longer-term outcome will be that she's not frustrated at the other person or at herself.

Requests for your input, time, or energy will elicit a reaction in you of feeling either deflated, flattered, and excited or fairly neutral. If you've bought yourself time with the holding response, you can use it to revisit your values and assess whether this request takes you toward a value or away from one. The pause allows time for your nervous system to settle so you're not making a knee-jerk response.

Benefits of Boundaries

As you start to choose healthy options, this will start to set expectations of what you will and won't do and how quickly you will get to something. For example, if others know that you only do emailing for an hour, once a day, they'll get accustomed to your responses taking twenty-four hours. This means it will get easier for you to make this choice in the future, as you are training the people around you to honor your boundaries.

You will also be modeling healthy boundaries to others. We talked about rest as a form of rebellion in Chapter 7; here we go one step further with boundaries as a form of activism!

Find Your Tribe

To help you on your journey, you will also benefit from finding your "tribe"—others who are on the same path to committing to self-care and boundary setting. Then you won't need to keep explaining your choices and you'll have people around you who will celebrate your decisions to oppose burnout culture. Tell others that you're working on reducing your burnout by managing your boundaries and invite them to join you.

Be rebels who rest and say "No" together!

What Next with Boundaries?

Boundaries are such a big topic and so important. Keep in mind that you will need to continually tend to them. Think of your boundaries as a wooden fence around you, and the external pressures and cultural norms are the winds constantly battering it. You will need to consciously keep working to maintain your fence.

LOOSEN UP HIGH STANDARDS

Perfectionists often set themselves unrelenting high standards: These are expectations of a level of achievement so high, they cannot possibly reach it all the time or only at a huge cost, such as overworking, being hard on themselves, or putting off starting things until they can do them perfectly (procrastination).

When the standard isn't reached, a perfectionist concludes that they didn't try hard enough or that they are a failure instead of assessing how helpful or realistic the standard was in the first place. For example, if you're a student, your unrelenting high standard could be that you're always in the top 5 percent of your class; or if you're a business owner, you aspire to customer-service excellence such that there are no unhappy customers or refund requests.

How to Reset Your Standards

- If you haven't yet done so, go back to Chapter 8 and map out your burnout backstory to get a sense of how your self-worth is tied to the need to achieve. This will give you insight as to why you currently set such high standards. The post-burnout-growth opportunity here is to consider how helpful these standards are in living according to your values (see Chapter 13) for a full and meaningful life. They may serve you in a very narrow way, such as being at the top of the league table for hitting targets or having a perfect attendance record. But is the cost of burnout worth it? Write two lists: one of the things you'll be sacrificing if you let go of these high standards and one of the things you'll gain and why that's important to you.

- Reflect on other domains of life from Chapter 12 that give you a sense of self-worth aside from achieving gold standards in one narrow area, such as education or work. The exercise in Chapter 13 for reconnecting with your values (see page 220) will be helpful in reminding you what else is important and will allow you to broaden out your focus from the narrow attention on one area.

- The first two steps are about helping you become more motivated to change your standards. It can be scary to do things differently, and the likelihood is that you will notice worrisome thoughts popping up around failing or being thought of negatively when you start to lower your standards. In therapy, we call this a leap of faith. You logically know that you will benefit from a practical change, but doing it feels anxiety-provoking. So start very small. Test out what it's like to tweak your standards just a little to fit better with your well-being. For example, what if you go home ten minutes earlier or only clean up five of the kids' toys in the evening rather than tidying the whole room? Can you have a pizza night rather than a home-prepared meal? Or, as in Suraj's case, could you tell the client that revisions will now take an extra day so you don't need to drop everything to do them?

- Make a decision about how long to try this out for (two weeks, for example), then come back and evaluate. Make a note of your main worry now. Perhaps it's that your boss will be annoyed, you'll fall behind with coursework, or you'll be overlooked for opportunities. When you evaluate your new standards, check in with these worries and whether they came true or not. You can also check in with the other domains of your life and ask yourself whether you feel more aligned with your values and, if so, how you can recognize this.

REDISCOVER JOY

One of the big losses in burnout is joy. Joy is a positive (green mode) emotion. It is felt when we are engaged with something that is good for us—often activities that involve exploration, filling up on resources, and connection (which allowed our ancestors to make helpful discoveries and seek out food, a mate, and friendship). Joy occurs through positive stimulation of the senses, whether through listening to an uplifting song, creative pastimes, seeing your favorite comedian on TV, sharing a moment of closeness with a friend, or simply tasting a delicious slice of chocolate cake.

One way of rediscovering joy is to find ways to be playful. Many adults forget how to play or fail to see the value in it. Play can come from activities like creativity, socializing, music, and exercise.

What types of things used to give you joy that you've stopped doing? Go as far back as you can even if it seems silly—that's part of the importance of this reflection. Are there creative, sporty, or musical activities that you could try picking up again? What types of things have surprised you with a burst of joy and how can you do more of them? Here are some personal examples of joy that surprised me recently: a short burst of running with my youngest child to get to the play area; seeing a feather-shaped cloud float by; watching my guinea pigs tussle over their hay.

Choose one area to focus on at a time. Change is hard, so go slowly. If you can access therapy, this can play a role in various ways with burnout recovery, including making lasting changes. Talking therapies that might help include cognitive behavioral therapy (CBT) which can assist with boundaries, getting familiar with your anxiety triggers, working on your perfectionist standards, and practicing assertiveness; and EMDR which can help you process any blocks to self-care or healthy boundaries, especially when they've come from past traumas. I've referred a few times to the merits of mindfulness, ACT (see page 220), and CFT (see page 165), all of which are very helpful in going deeper with the themes in this book. Finally, you might consider coaching to get accountability and support in making practical changes to your work or business. You can get coaching for many areas, such as life, parenting, business, and so on. Used in conjunction with the tools outlined in this chapter, these therapies can really set you up for success.

FINAL THOUGHTS

MOST PEOPLE WHO have become burned out know there are healthy habits they should be practicing to care for themselves during high-stress periods, but they struggle to actually do them. My main objective in writing this book has been to help you get out of your own way by understanding the internal pressures that currently stop you from acting in your own best interests.

Remember that the environment you are in will not suddenly stop being stressful, busy, and overstimulating; in other words, your threat system will continue to react. So your recovery from burnout is likely going on within the harmful context that created the difficulties in the first place. This means that your nervous system will continue to be bombarded by messages to react quickly and to strive to retain your place in society. The steps in this book give you the guidance for taking mini-everyday respite from this and for leaning into the reminders of connection and safety. This will be easier at some times than at others; recovery is a bumpy road. Here is what I draw out for my therapy clients when we have a final session:

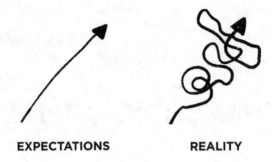

EXPECTATIONS   **REALITY**

When you hit a low or feel like you're back in the old, unhealthy patterns, know that this is normal and to be expected. Your inner critic will have a field day at moments like this, telling you you've failed and that change is impossible. But please remember that you are not back at square one, because you now have psychological insight, reflections on your personal patterns, and tools at your disposal for support.

The human nervous system is an amazing biological piece of equipment, always watching out for you and there to support you through emergencies. But all too often, we aren't taught about this part of being human. Nor are we taught how to nurture this system so that it can support us in the best way possible through life's stresses.

This book has given you the insight you need to strengthen your ability to move through your nervous-system gears so that you can quiet the stress and anxiety. Keep it close by so you can dip into it to remind yourself how to get back on track whenever you need to. And I hope that it will serve you well.

REFERENCES

INTRODUCTION
Page xiii: "Burnout is 'a disease of civilization',…"
Chabot, P. (2018). *Global Burnout.* London: Bloomsbury.

Page xiv: "…or label them with an anxiety or depression disorder instead."
van Dam, A. (2021). A clinical perspective on burnout: diagnosis, classification, and treatment of clinical burnout. *European Journal of Work and Organizational Psychology, 30*(5), 732–741.

Page xv: "…'second shift' the moment you get home from work…"
Hochschild, A. and Machung, A. (2012). *The Second Shift: Working Families and the Revolution at Home.* New York, NY: Penguin Books.

Page xv: "…research shows that females often end up doing the lion's share…"
Bianchi, S., Sayer, L. C., Milkie, M. A., and Robinson, J. R. (2012). Housework: who did, does or will do it, and how much does it matter? *Social Forces, 91,* 55–63.

Page xvi: "polyvagal theory"
Porges, S. W. (2011). *The Polyvagal Theory.* New York/London: W. W. Norton & Company.

Porges, S. W. (2017). *The Pocket Guide to the Polyvagal Theory.* New York/London: W. W. Norton & Company.

Page xvii: "…compassion-focused therapy…"
Gilbert, P. (2010). *The Compassionate Mind (Compassion Focused Therapy).* London: Robinson.

REFERENCES

CHAPTER 1

Page 6: "Data from the Sydney studies."
Parker, G., Tavella, G., and Eyers, K. (2022). *Burnout: A Guide to Identifying Burnout and Pathways to Recovery*. London: Routledge.

Tavella, G., Hadzi-Pavlovic, D., and Parker, G. (2020). Burnout: re-examining its key constructs. *Psychiatry Research, 287*.

Page 8: "...Barry Farber into therapist and teacher burnout led to findings that..."
Farber, B. (1990). Burnout in psychotherapists: incidence, types, and trends. *Psychotherapy in Private Practice*. 8, 35–44. 10.1300/J294v08n01_07.

Montero-Marín, J., García-Campayo, J., Mera, D. M., and del Hoyo, Y. L. (2009). A new definition of burnout syndrome based on Farber's proposal. *Journal of Occupational Medicine and Toxicology, 4*(31).

Page 11: "Research into parental temperament suggests..."
Piotrowski, K., Bojanowska, A., Szczygieł, D., Mikolajczak, M., and Roskam, I. (2023). Parental burnout at different stages of parenthood: links with temperament, big five traits, and parental identity. *Frontiers in Psychology, 14*.

Page 11: "The burden of caring..."
Alzheimer's Association (2024). Special report: mapping a better future for dementia care navigation. *Alzheimer's disease facts and figures*. www.alz.org/media/Documents/alzheimers-facts-and-figures.pdf.

Page 11: "Research in Poland that surveyed the needs of informal care-givers of dependents..."
Szlenk-Czyczerska, E., Guzek, M., Bielska, D. E., Ławnik, A., Polanski, P., and Kurpas, D. (2020). Needs, aggravation, and degree of burnout in informal caregivers of patients with chronic cardiovascular disease. *International Journal of Environmental Research and Public Health, 17*.

Page 12: "...with rates of burnout ranging from 7.3 percent to 75.2 percent..."
Ilić, I. M. and Ilić, M. D. (2023). The relationship between the burnout syndrome and academic success of medical students: a cross-sectional study. *Archives of Industrial Hygiene and Toxicology, 74*(2), 134–141.

Page 12: "...For example, they may make more demands of their team..."
Parent-Lamarche, A. and Biron, C. (2022). When bosses are burned

out: psychosocial safety climate and its effect on managerial quality. *International Journal of Stress Management, 29*(3), 219–228.

Page 13: "...in entrepreneurial burnout is having autonomy..."
Tahar, Y. B., Rejeb, N., Maalaoui, A., Kraus, S., Westhead, P., and Jones, P. (2023). Emotional demands and entrepreneurial burnout: the role of autonomy and job satisfaction. *Small Business Economics, 61*, 701–716.

Page 14: "There are numerous studies showing how our organs..."
McEwen, B. (2000). Allostasis and allostatic load: implications for neuropsychopharmacology. *Neuropsychopharmacology, 22*, 108–124.

Page 14: "...are a few examples of physical ailments."
Salvagioni, D. A. J., Melanda, F. N., Mesas, A. E., Gonzalez, A. D., Gabani, F. L., and de Andrade, S. M. (2017). Physical, psychological and occupational consequences of job burnout: a systematic review of prospective studies. *PLoS ONE 12*(10).

Page 16: "Depression is an experience generally brought on by difficult life events..."
Bowden, G., Holltum, S., Shankar, R., Cooke, A., and Kinderman, P. (eds) (2020). *Understanding Depression. Why Adults Experience Depression and What Can Help.* British Psychological Society (Division of Clinical Psychology).

Page 17: "Research shows low testosterone in men can lead to fatigue, low mood, and insomnia."
Rivas, A. M., Mulkey, Z., Lado-Abeal, J., and Yarbrough, S. (2014). Diagnosing and managing low serum testosterone. *Proceedings (Baylor University. Medical Center), 27*(4), 321–324.

Page 17: "Maslach Burnout Inventory (MBI)..."
https://www.mindgarden.com/ (an online psychological assessment website for burnout measures).

Page 18: "Copenhagen Burnout Inventory (CBI)..."
Kristensen, T. S., Borritz, M., Villadsen, E., and Christensen, K. B. (2005). The Copenhagen burnout inventory: a new tool for the assessment of burnout. *Work & Stress, 19*(3), 192–207.

Page 18: "Parental Burnout Assessment (PBA)..."
Roskam, I., Bayot, M., and Mikolajczak, M. (2022). Parental Burnout

Assessment (PBA). In: Medvedev, O. N., Krägeloh, C. U., Siegert, R. J., and Singh, N. N. (eds). (2024). *Handbook of Assessment in Mindfulness Research*. Springer.

Page 18: "Informal Caregiver Burnout Inventory (ICB-10)…"
James, N. (2020). Rethinking burnout in informal caregivers: development and validation of the informal caregiver burnout inventory—10 item form. *Electronic Theses and Dissertations, 369*.

Page 20: "The Five Stages of Burnout"
Veninga, R. Work, stress and health. Four major conclusions. *Occupational Health Nursing*, June 1982.

Veninga, R. and Spradley, J. P. (1981). *The Work/Stress Connection: How to Cope with Job Burnout*. Boston: Little, Brown.

Page 23: "…make them they are less rational…"
Michailidis, E. and Banks, A. P. (2016). The relationship between burnout and risk-taking in workplace decision-making and decision-making style. *Work & Stress, 30*(3), 278–292.

Page 23: "…more likely to compare yourself unfavorably to others…"
Buunk, A. P. and Brenninkmeijer, V. (2022). Burnout, social comparison orientation and the responses to social comparison among teachers in the Netherlands. *International Journal of Environmental Research and Public Health, 19*(20).

Page 25: "…an average of one to three years…"
Bernier, D. (1998). A study of coping: successful recovery from severe burnout and other reactions to severe work-related stress. *Work & Stress, 12*(1), 50–65.

Page 25: "…at the mid to lower end of the continnum…"
Mäkikangas, A., Leiter, M. P., Kinnunen, U., and Feldt, T. (2021). Profiling development of burnout over eight years: relation with job demands and resources. *European Journal of Work and Organizational Psychology, 30*(5), 720–731.

Page 27: "Neuroticism is a personality trait that…"
Bianchi, R. (2018). Burnout is more strongly linked to neuroticism than to work-contextualized factors. *Psychiatry Research, 270*, 901–905.

REFERENCES

CHAPTER 2

Page 38: "Yerkes–Dodson Law"
Yerkes, R. M. and Dodson, J. D. (1908). The relation of strength of stimulus to rapidity of habit-formation. *Journal of Comparative Neurology and Psychology, 18*(5), 459–482.

Page 39: "In one experiment carried out by profesor of psychology at University of Virginia, Timothy Wilson, and colleagues in 2014…"
Wilson, T. D., Reinhard, D. A., Westgate E. C., Gilbert, D. T., Ellerbeck, N., Hahn, C., Brown, C. L., and Shaked, A. (2014). Just think: the challenges of the disengaged mind. *Science, 345,* 75–77.

Page 42: "…nowadays, we have social media telling us…"
Royal Society for Public Health publication (2017). *Social Media and Young People's Mental Health and Well-Being.*

Page 43: "…build-up referred to as the allostatic load…"
Guidi, J., Lucente, M., Sonino, N., and Fava, G. A. (2021). Allostatic load and its impact on health: a systematic review. *Psychotherapy and psychosomatics, 90*(1), 11–27.

Page 43: "…is the threat-response region, the amygdala…"
Zhang, X., Ge, T. T., Yin, G., Cui, R., Zhao, G., and Yang, W. (2018). Stress-induced functional alterations in amygdala: implications for neuropsychiatric diseases. *Frontiers in Neuroscience, 12,* 367.

Page 44: "Wounds take longer to heal…"
Marucha, P. T., Kiecolt-Glaser, J. K., and Favagehi, M. (1998). Mucosal wound healing is impaired by examination stress. *Psychosomatic Medicine, 60*(3), 362–365.

Page 44: "…experience problems with the gut like IBS."
Hod, K., Melamed, S., Dekel, R., Maharshak, N., and Sperber, A. D. (2020). Burnout, but not job strain, is associated with irritable bowel syndrome in working adults. *Journal of Psychosomatic Research, 134.*

Page 45: "…on our ability to focus and make decisions."
Harrison, Y. and Horne, J. A. (2000). The impact of sleep deprivation on decision making: a review. *Journal of Experimental Psychology: Applied, 6*(3), 236–249.

Page 46: Box: Using alcohol to unwind at the end of the day
Angarita, G., Emaldi, N., Hodges, S., Morgan., P. (2016). Sleep

abnormalities associated with alcohol, cannabis, cocaine, and opiate use: a comprehensive review. *Addiction Science and Clinical Practice*, 11, 9.

Page 48: "Gabor Maté defines trauma not as what happens to you..."
Mate, G. with Mate, D., (2022). *The Myth of Normal*. Vermillion, Ebury, London: Penguin Random House.

Page 50: "Trauma is what happens to a person where there is too much too soon, too much for too long, or not enough for too long."
Duros, P. and Crowley, D. (2014). The body comes to therapy too. *Clinical Social Work J* 42, 237–246.

Page 51: "...human distress Mary Boyle and Lucy Johnstone summarize the core human needs..."
Boyle, M. and Johnstone, L. (2020). *A Straight Talking Introduction to the Power Threat Meaning Framework: An Alternative to Psychiatric Diagnosis*. Monmouth, UK: PCCS Books.

Page 53: "Trauma is not what happens to us..."
Levine, P. A. (1997). *Waking the Tiger: Healing Trauma*. Berkley, California: North Atlantic Books.

Page 55: "...famous experiment was carried out by psychologist..."
Maier, S. F. and Seligman, M. E. (1976). Learned helplessness: theory and evidence. *Journal of Experimental Psychology: General*, 105, 3–46.

Page 56: "The origin of trauma is the inability to move..."
Van der Kolk, B. (2014). *The Body Keeps the Score*. New York: Viking Penguin.

CHAPTER 3
Page 61: "Brain scans show that a surprising amount of activity occurs..."
Raichle, M. E., Macleon A. M., Synder, A. Z., et al. (2001). A default mode of brain function. *Proceedings of the National Academy of Sciences of the United States*, 98, 676–682.

Page 65: "Procedural memory is housed deep inside the brain (the basal ganglia)..."
Yin, H. and Knowlton, B. (2006). The role of the basal ganglia in habit formation. *Nature Reviews Neuroscience*, 7, 464–476.

CHAPTER 4

Page 73: "…we can experiment with glimmers."
Dana, D. (2020). *Polyvagal Exercises for Safety and Connection.* New York/London: W. W. Norton & Company. Boulder, Colorado: Sounds True.

Page 75: "Our sensory systems prefer stimuli from the natural…"
Wilson, E. O. (2007). Biophilia and the conservation ethic. In: Penn, D. J. and Mysterud, I. (eds). *Evolutionary Perspectives on Environmental Problems.* London: Routledge.

Coburn, A., Vartanian, O., and Chatterjee, A. (2014). Buildings, beauty, and the brain: a neuroscience of architectural experience. *Journal of Cognitive Neuroscience, 29,* 1521–1530.

Page 77: "Research now shows this left-right, bilateral movement allows us to stay alert…"
Salay, L. D., Ishiko, N., and Huberman, A. D. (2018). A midline thalamic circuit determines reactions to visual threat. *Nature, 557,* 183–189.

De Voogd, L. D., Kanen, J. W., Neville, D. A., Roelofs, K., Fernandez, G., and Hermans, E. J. (2018). Eye-movement intervention enhances extinction via amygdala deactivation. *Journal of Neuroscience, 38,* 8694–8706.

Page 79: "Blue spaces like coastlines and rivers improve…"
Bell, S., Phoenix, C., Lovell, R., and Wheeler, B. (2015). Seeking every-day well-being: the coast as a therapeutic landscape. *Social Sciences and Medicine, 142,* 56–67.

Page 79: "…improves the effects of stress linked to technology anxiety."
Wen, Y., Yan, Q., Pan, Y. et al. (2019). Medical empirical research on forest bathing (*Shinrin-yoku*): a systematic review. *Environmental Health and Preventative Medicine, 24,* 70.

Page 79: "…spending just ninety seconds looking at an image of forests has a calming effect on subjects' physiologies."
Song, C., Ikei, H., and Mikazaki, Y., (2018). Physiological effects of visual stimulation with forest imagery. *International Journal of Environmental Research and Public Health, 15,* 213.

Page 80: "Keza MacDonald publicly shared how her escape into video game…"

Macdonald, K. (2020). Video games can improve mental health: let's stop seeing them as a guilty pleasure. www.theguardian.com/comment isfree/2020/nov/23/video-games-boost-mental-health-stop-guilty -pleasure.

Page 82: "You can see this in videos of development psychologist Edward Tronick's still-face experiment…"
Weinberg, M. K., Beeghly, M., Olson, K. L., and Tronick, E. (2008). A still-face paradigm for young children: 2½ year-olds' reactions to maternal unavailability during the still-face. *The Journal of Developmental Processes, 3*(1), 4–22.

Page 82: "The good news is that low vagal tone can improve with…"
Rockliff, H., Gilbert, P., Mcewan, K., Lightman, S., and Glover, D. (2008). A pilot exploration of heart rate variability and salivary cortisol responses to compassion-focused imagery. *Clinical Neuropsychiatry, 5*(3), 132–139.

Page 84: "According to Gartner, a technology company providing research and advisory data…"
Stamford, C. (2020). Gartner says worldwide end-user spending on cloud-based web conferencing solutions will grow nearly 25% in 2020, *Gartner* online article: www.gartner.com/en/newsroom/press-releases /2020-06-02-gartner-says-worldwide-end-user-spending-on -cloud-based-web-conferencing-solutions-will-grow-nearly-25-per cent-in-2020.

Page 84: "This coincides with increased reports of Zoom fatigue…"
Bullock, A., Colvin, A., and Jackson, S. (2021). "All Zoomed out": strategies for addressing Zoom fatigue in the age of COVID-19. In: *Innovations in Learning and Technology for the Workplace and Higher Education.* 61–68. Switzerland: Springer Nature.

Page 84: "Research into the reason for this highlights: overly intense eye…"
Doring. N., Moor, K., Fielder, M., Schoenenberg. K., and Raake, A. (2022). Videoconference fatigue: a conceptual analysis. *Inter-national Journal of Environmental Research and Public Health, 19,* 2061.

Karl, K. A., Peluchette, J. V., and Aghakhani, N. (2022). Virtual work meetings during the COVID-19 pandemic: the good, bad, and ugly. *Small Group Research, 53*(3), 343–365.

REFERENCES

Page 85: "…on social media in their lifetime…"
Average daily time spent on social media (Latest 2024 data): https://www.broadbandsearch.net/blog/average-daily-time-on-social-media.

Page 85: "…but, in the words of Deb Dana, …"
Dana. D. (2018). *The Polyvagal Theory in Therapy.* New York/London: W. W. Norton & Company.

Page 85: "In January 2023, an article in The New York Times…"
Dunn, J. (2023). Day 2: the secret power of the 8-minute telephone call. *New York Times* online. https://www.nytimes.com/2023/01/02/well/phone-call-happiness-challenge.html

Page 85: "followed by an exploration of this in Stylist *magazine."*
Crockett, M. (2023). https://www.stylist.co.uk/relationships/family-friends/power-of-an-8-minute-phone-call/761827.

Page 85: "A 2022 survey by the UK Office of National Statistics…"
Facts and statistics to end loneliness. Article on the Campaign to End Loneliness website (a Community Interest Company). https://www.campaigntoendloneliness.org/facts-and-statistics.

Page 85: "Within the workplace, America's most lonely professions are…"
Achor, S., Kellerman, G. R., Reece, A., and Robichaux, A. (2018). America's loneliest workers, according to research. *Harvard Business Review.* (hbr.org) https://hbr.org/2018/03/americas-loneliest-workers-according-to-research.

Page 89: "In a 2001 study in California, shopper behavior was observed…"
Iyengar, S. and Lepper, M. (2001). When choice is demotivating: can one desire too much of a good thing? *Journal of Personality and Social Psychology,* 79(6), 995–1006.

Page 89: "Beth Berry gives examples of the…"
Berry, B. (2020). *Motherwhelmed.* Revolution from Home Publishing.

CHAPTER 5
Page 97: "…neck area where research shows it has the strongest impact on heart rate…"
Jungmann, M., Vencatachellum, S., Van Ryckeghem, D., and Vögele, C.

(2018). Effects of cold stimulation on cardiac-vagal activation in healthy participants: randomized controlled trial. *JMIR Formative Research*, 2(2), 10257.

Page 101: "...which a 2023 study showed to be one of the quickest..."
Balban, M. Y., Neri, E., Kogon, M. M., Weed, L., Nouriani, B., Jo, B., Holl, G., Zeitzer, J. M., Spiegel, D., and Huberman, A. D. (2023). Brief structured respiration practices enhance mood and reduce physiological arousal. *Cell Reports Medicine*, 4(1).

Page 105: "...Eye Movement Desensitization and Reprocessing..."
Shapiro. F. (2018). *Eye Movement Desensitization and Reprocessing (EMDR) Therapy, Basic Principles, Protocol and Procedures*. London: The Guildford Press.

Page 110: "Regular yoga practice has been shown to have a stronger..."
Streeter, C. C., Whitfield, T. H., Owen, L., Rein, T., Karri, S. K., Yakhkind, A., Perlmutter, R., Prescot, A., Renshaw, P. F., Ciraulo, D. A., and Jensen, J. E. (2010). Effects of yoga versus walking on mood, anxiety, and brain GABA levels: a randomized controlled MRS study. *Journal of Alternative and Complementary Medicine*, 16(11), 1145–1152.

Page 111: "There is emerging evidence that this can support people who meet..."
Kuhfuß, M., Maldei, T., Hetmanek, A., and Baumann, N. (2021). Somatic experiencing—effectiveness and key factors of a body-oriented trauma therapy: a scoping literature review. *European Journal of Psychotraumatology*, 12(1).

CHAPTER 6
Page 119: "...access to fewer healthy skills in self-soothing."
Lieter, M. P., Day, A., and Price, L. (2015). Attachment styles at work: measurement, collegial relationships, and burnout. *Burnout Research*, 2(1), 25–35.

Page 120: "People with this attachment style are more likely to get overly involved in work..."
Hardy, G. E. and Barkham, M. (1994). The relationship between interpersonal attachment styles and work difficulties. *Human Relations*, 47(3), 263–281.

Page 121: "...which compassion expert Paul Gilbert calls..."
Gilbert, P., Broomhead, C., Irons, C., McEwan, K., Bellew, R., Mills, A.,

Gale, C., and Knibb, R. (2007). Development of a striving to avoid inferiority scale. *Br J Soc Psychol*, *46*(Pt 3), 633–648.

Page 121: "...even in situations where someone logically knows..."
Asa, N., Kenichi, A., and Yasuhiro, K. (2022). Moderating effects of striving to avoid inferiority on income and mental health. *Frontiers in Psychology*, *13*.

Page 126: "in 1998 with researcher and psychology professor Benjamin Dykman..."
Dykman, B. M. (1998). Integrating cognitive and motivational factors in depression: initial tests of a goal-orientation approach. *Journal of Personality and Social Psychology*, *74*(1), 139–158.

Page 128: "...where an eldest child is likely to be high achieving..."
Paulhus, D. L., Trapnell, P. D., and Chen, D. (1999). Birth order effects on personality and achievement within families. *Psychological Science*, *10*(6), 482–488.

CHAPTER 7
Page 133: "Research carried out by social psychologist..."
Maslach, C. and Leiter, M. P. (2016). Understanding the burnout experience: recent research and its implications for psychiatry. *World Psychiatry*, *15*(2), 103–111.

Page 136: "An article in the Journal of Nursing Scholarship *considered..."*
Stokes-Parish, J., Elliott, R., Rolls, K., and Massey, D. (2020). Angels and heroes: the unintended consequence of the hero narrative. *Journal of Nursing Scholarship*, *52*(5), 462–466.

Page 136: "...62 percent of nursing staff report burnout..."
Schmidt, A. (2020). We need to talk about burnout the same way we do about benefits. American Hospital Association. https://www.aha.org/news/blog/2020-10-20-we-need-talk-about-burnout-same-way-we-talk-about-benefits.

Page 137: "Professor Kenneth V. Hardy (from the couple and family..."
Hardy, K. (2013). Healing the hidden wounds of racial trauma. *Reclaiming Children and Youth*, *22*, 24–28.

Page 138: "...the Nagoski sisters link this to the concept of human-giver syndrome..."
Nagoski, E. and Nagoski, A. (2020). *Burnout: Solve Your Stress Cycle*. Vermillion, Ebury, London: Penguin Random House.

REFERENCES

Page 142: "Situational factors that skew this natural comparison process..."
Garcia, S. M., Tor, A., and Schiff, T. M. (2013). The psychology of competition: a social comparison perspective. *Perspectives on Psychological Science,* 8(6), 634–650.

Page 143: "But burned-out individuals are more likely to interpret this type of comparison negatively..."
Buunk, A. P. and Brenninkmeijer, V. (2022). Burnout, social comparison orientation and the responses to social comparison among teachers in the Netherlands. *International journal of Environmental Research and Public Health,* 19(20).

CHAPTER 8

Page 149: "There are three types of perfectionist, the first two of..."
Smith, M. M., Saklofske, D. H., Stoeber, J., and Sherry, S. B. (2016). The big three perfectionism scale: a new measure of perfectionism. *Journal of Psychoeducational Assessment,* 34(7), 670–687.

Page 152: "Emma Reed Turrell, author of Please Yourself..."
Turrell, E. R. (2021). *Please Yourself: How to Stop People-Pleasing & Transform the Way You Live.* London: 4th Estate.

CHAPTER 9

Page 164: "People with unhealthy levels of perfectionism..."
Pereira, A. T., Brito, M. A., Cabacos, C., Carneiro, M., Calvalho, F., Manao, A., Araujo, A., Pereria, D., and Macedo, A. (2022). The protective role of self-compassion in the relationship between perfectionism and burnout in portuguese medicine and dentistry students. *International Journal of Environmental Research and Public Health, Special Issue: Academic and Emotional Determinants of Perfectionism,* 19, 2740.

Page 164: "A study in 2016 discovered that people who struggle to show themselves self-compassion tend..."
Hermanto, N. and Zuroff, D. (2016). The social mentality theory of self-compassion and self-reassurance: the interactive effect of care-seeking and caregiving. *The Journal of Social Psychology,* 156(5), 523–535.

Page 165: "...three systems of emotions regulation..."
Gilbert, P. (2009). *The Compassionate Mind (Compassion Focused Therapy).* London: Robinson.

REFERENCES

CHAPTER 10

Page 174: "...who are autistic or meet the criteria for ADHD..."
Wiersema, J. R. and Godefroid, E. (2018). Interoceptive awareness in attention deficit hyperactivity disorder. *PLoS ONE, 13*(10), e0205221.

Page 187: "There is a lot of research that shows that mindfulness..."
Goodman, M. J. and Schorling, J. B. (2012). A mindfulness course decreases burnout and improves well-being among healthcare providers. *Int J Psychiatry Med, 43*(2):119–128.

Page 187: "...reduction (MBSR) framework demonstrating consistently good evidence..."
Kriakous, S. A., Elliott, K. A., Lamers, C., and Owen, R. (2021). The effectiveness of mindfulness-based stress reduction on the psychological functioning of healthcare professionals: a systematic review. *Mindfulness, 12*(1), 1–28.

Page 187: "Mindfulness is also incorporated into other therapy approaches like CFT..."
Eriksson, T., Germundsjö, L., Åström, E., and Rönnlund, M. (2018). Mindful self-compassion training reduces stress and burnout symptoms among practicing psychologists: a randomized controlled trial of a brief web-based intervention. *Frontiers in Psychology, 9.*

Page 187: "...and acceptance and commitment therapy (ACT)..."
Towey-Swift, K. D., Lauvrud, C., and Whittington, R. (2023). Acceptance and commitment therapy (ACT) for professional staff burnout: a systematic review and narrative synthesis of controlled trials. *Journal of Mental Health, 32*(2), 452–464.

CHAPTER 11

Page 189: "It has been shown to improve..."
Luo, X., Qiao, L., and Che, X. (2018). Self-compassion modulates heart rate variability and negative affect to experimentally induced stress. *Mindfulness, 9*, 1522–1528.

Page 192: "The following table is a model from The Compassionate Mind Workbook..."
Irons, C. and Beaumont. E. (2017). *The Compassionate Mind Workbook*. London: Robinson.

Page 198: "Gratitude practices have been shown..."
Regan, A., Walsh, L. C., and Lyubomirsky, S. (2023). Are some ways of expressing gratitude more beneficial than others? Results from a randomized controlled experiment. *Affective Science, 4*, 72–81.

Page 198: "...our social-engagement circuitry lights up..."
Fox, G. R., Kaplan, J., Damasio, H., and Damasio, A. (2015). Neural correlates of gratitude. *Frontiers in Psychology, 6.*

Page 198: "A study where coworkers were asked to write..."
Hori, D., Sasahara, S., Doki, S., Oi, Y., and Matsuzaki, I. (2020). Prefrontal activation while listening to a letter of gratitude read aloud by a coworker face-to-face: a NIRS study. *PLoS ONE, 15*(9), e0238715.

Page 199: "Fortunately, a 2015 study led by Joel Wong showed..."
Wong, Y. J., Owen, J., Gabana, N. T., Brown, J. W., McInnis, S., Toth, P., and Gilman, L. (2018). Does gratitude writing improve the mental health of psychotherapy clients? Evidence from a randomized controlled trial. *Psychotherapy Research, 28*(2), 192–202.

Page 200: "You may have heard of the 'power pose'..."
Carney, D., Cuddy, A., and Yap, A. (2010). Power posing: brief nonverbal displays affect neuroendocrine levels and risk tolerance. *Psychological Science, 21*, 10.

Page 201: "Research by compassionate mind experts has built on..."
Gilbert, P., Basran, J. K., Plowright, P., and Gilbert, H. (2023). Energizing compassion: using music and community focus to stimulate compassion drive and sense of connectedness. *Frontier in Psychology, 14.*

CHAPTER 12

Page 203: "Research consistently shows that it protects from burnout, even in situations where..."
McEwan, K., Minou, L., Moore, H., and Gilbert, P. (2020). Engaging with distress: training in the compassionate approach. *Journal of Psychiatry and Mental Health Nursing, 27*(6), 718–727.

Page 207: "...five-to-one ratio..."
Gottman, J. and Levenson, R. (1992). Marital processes predictive of later dissolution: behavior, physiology and health. *Journal of Personality and Social Psychology, 63*, 221–233.

REFERENCES

Page 216: "Research suggests that about 50–70 percent…"
Wu, X., Kaminga, A. C., Dai, W., Deng, J., Wang, Z., Pan, X., and Liu, A. (2019). The prevalence of moderate-to-high posttraumatic growth: a systematic review and meta-analysis. *Journal of Affective Disorders, 243*, 408–415.

Page 216: "…who are open to reconsidering their belief systems…"
Collier, L. (2016). Growth after trauma: why are some people more resilient than others—and can it be taught? *Monitor on Psychology, 47*(10), 48.

CHAPTER 13

Page 220: "Have a look at the domains…"
Harris, R. https://thehappinesstrap.com/upimages/Values_Questionnaire .pdf.

Page 224: "Research shows that visualizing an outcome helps us…"
Ungerleider, S. and Golding, J. M. (1991). Mental practice among Olympic athletes. *Perceptual and Motor Skills, 72* (3 pt. 1), 1007–1017.

CHAPTER 14

Page 234: "…is from psychologist Suzy Reading in her book Rest to Reset*…"*
Reading, S. (2023). *Rest to Reset.* London: Aster.

Page 236: "Now, however, updated research suggests that not all screen time…"
Huiberts, L. M., Opperhuizen, A. L., and Schlangen, L. J. M. (2022). Pre-bedtime activities and light-emitting screen use in college students and their relationships with self-reported sleep duration and quality. *Lighting Research and Technology, 54*, 6.

ACKNOWLEDGMENTS

Thank you to everyone who has supported me with this project. Jen, my agent, you've been amazing. So patient and generous with your time. You are so good at breaking everything down into manageable chunks for me (and creating a Dropbox file for it!).

Everyone at Yellow Kite and Balance, particularly the acquisitions editors Carolyn and Renee, for believing in this book and bringing it to life, and to my copy editor Anne for your keen eye and skill.

Thank you to all the professionals whose research and models I've drawn on in this book, I hope I've done your concepts and ideas justice.

Thank you to the psychologists who read drafts or met with me to allow space to discuss ideas: Dr. Nancy Bancroft, Dr. Shelley Kerr, Dr. Jenny Weall, Prof. Paul Gilbert, Dr. Naomi Sams, Dr. Claire Husbands, Dr. Mia Hobbs, Dr. Sarah Butler, and everyone else in my associate practice, supervision groups, and my University of East London cohort where I had these conversations.

Thank you to my parents, siblings, family, and friends who have been so patient with me while I have worked on this. I've really appreciated your moral support when you've checked in with how it's going or cooked me a curry after a day of writing!

ACKNOWLEDGMENTS

Thank you to all my clients, past and present, who have allowed me to be part of their journeys and have inspired me in so many ways.

Thank you to my three children for being so enthusiastic about this book and telling everyone they know to buy a copy.

Finally, thank you to my wonderful husband for creating space for me to write by taking on the lion's share of life's duties, household chores, and childcare. Your belief in me and words of encouragement mean so much.

RESOURCES AND FURTHER READING

ACCESSING THERAPY

If you would like to consider working with a therapist using the models discussed in this book, I recommend utilizing these resources to find someone with the right training and accreditation:

Association for Behavioral and Cognitive Therapies for accredited CBT therapists: www.abct.org

Compassionate Mind Foundation's directory of therapists: www .cfttherapist.com

Eye Movement Desensitization and Reprocessing (EMDR) EMDRIA: www.emdria.org

Mindfulness Based Stress Reduction (MBSR): www.MBSRtraining .com

Association for Contextual Behavioral Science directory for an ACT trained therapist: www.contextualscience.org

Trauma Release Exercise (TRE®): www.traumaprevention.com

Somatic Experiencing®: www.traumahealing.org

GOING DEEPER WITH THEMES FROM THIS BOOK

Polyvagal Theory

Dana, D. (2021). *Anchored*. Colorado: Sounds True. A book by the therapist Deb Dana who has worked with Stephen Porges to make the concepts from polyvagal theory practical.

Porges, S. W. and Porges, S. (2023). *Our Polyvagal World*. New York: W. W. Norton & Co. Written by the originator of polyvagal theory and his brother. This explores the ways in which we can make certain environments like prisons, schools, and workplaces more user-friendly for our nervous systems to thrive.

TraumaGeek.com is run by researcher-storyteller Janae-Elisabeth. She has helpful blogs and essays that interpret everyday life and issues related to neurodivergence through a Polyvagal lens.

Supportive Apps

HeartMath: A biofeedback app with a course to learn how to regulate yourself. Check out their website for more information: www.heartmath.com.

The Self Compassion App: This app was built by two leading experts in compassionate mind therapy, which includes a course, meditations, and also a biofeedback tool.

Habit Tracker: An easy-to-use app for building good habits in your self-care.

Freedom: An app for managing your phone usage, helpful for reducing stimulation during your wind down routine if you tend to multi-task on your phone.

Self-Assessment Tools

The Strive to Avoid Inferiority scale is freely available online and can help you identify areas of competitiveness or concerns that lead to unhealthy striving or achieving behaviors. Locate it at www.compassionatemind.co.uk.

The Big Three Perfectionism Scale is a helpful tool for assessing your perfectionism type. Smith, M. M., Saklofske, D. H., Stoeber, J., and Sherry, S. B. (2016). The big three perfectionism scale: a new measure of perfectionism. *Journal of Psychoeducational Assessment*.

More Help for People-Pleasing

Glover Tawwab, N. (2021). *Set Boundaries, Find Peace: A Guide to Reclaiming Yourself*. New York: TarcherPerigee. An accessible and comprehensive guide to the areas of your life where boundaries are needed and practical scripts and wording to start setting these.

Turrell, E. R. (2021). *Please Yourself. How to Stop People Pleasing and & Transform the Way You Live*. London: 4th Estate, HarperCollins.

A helpful book written by a therapist showing the various ways you might people-please and how to address it in the various areas of life (friendships, work, and family).

Assert Yourself! A free workbook is available on the Center for Clinical Interventions' website: www.cci.health.wa.gov.au/Resources/Looking-After-Yourself/Assertiveness.

More Help for Perfectionism

Overcome Perfectionism. A free workbook is available on the Center for Clinical Interventions' website: https://www.cci.health.wa.gov.au/Resources/Looking-After-Yourself/Perfectionism.

Kemp, J. and Coyne, L. (2022). *The ACT Workbook for Perfectionism.* New Harbinger. The go-to resource for ACT-trained therapists working with perfectionism in therapy.

Pause, Purpose, Play podcast. Hosted by psychologist Michaela Thomas with therapy tips and interviews aimed at high-achieving, perfectionist females in danger of burning out.

More Help for Improving Your Relationship with Negative Emotions

Gilbert, P. (2009). *The Compassionate Mind.* Robinson, Little Brown. The original text for introducing the compassionate mind model by the creator of this approach.

Irons, C. and Beaumont, E. (2017). *The Compassionate Mind Workbook.* Robinson, Little Brown. Practical guidance through the compassionate mind approach. Each chapter breaks down the concepts so you can work through them and the exercises.

Kolts, R. (2012). *The Compassionate Mind Approach to Managing Your Anger.* Robinson. A deep dive into anger from a member of the compassionate mind team. Learn more clearly about the purpose of your anger and compassionate ways of responding.

Facing Your Feelings. A free workbook is available on the Center for Clinical Interventions' website: https://www.cci.health.wa.gov.au/Resources/Looking-After-Yourself/Tolerating-Distress.

Resources for Improving Self-Care

Clear, J. (2018). *Atomic Habits: An Easy and Proven Way to Build Health Habits and Break Bad Ones.* Penguin Random House. A popular book that gives a framework for improving everyday habits, from healthy eating to exercise.

Harris, R. (2007). *The Happiness Trap: Stop Struggling and Start Living*. Shambhala. Dr. Russ Harris is a leading expert in acceptance and commitment therapy. This book breaks down the concepts and has techniques to work through.

Nagoski, E. and Nagsoki, A. (2020). *Burnout: Solve Your Stress Cycle*. New York: Ballatine Books. A popular book aimed at females explaining how stress is experienced differently by them and contains practical ideas for managing stressors.

Reading, S. (2023). *Rest to Reset*. London: Aster. One of several books by Suzy Reading that gives practical and bite-size advice from her experience as a yoga teacher and psychologist.

Russell, T. (2017). *#What Is Mindfulness?* Watkins. Experienced neuroscientist and mindfulness teacher Tamara Russell introduces mindfulness in a really accessible way while linking it to neuroscience to help us understand it.

Parnell, L. (2008). *Tapping In: A Step by Step Guide to Activating Your Healing Resources Through Bilateral Simulation*. Boulder, Colorado: Sounds True.

Williams, M. and Penman, D. (2011). *Mindfulness: A Practical Guide to Finding Peace in a Frantic World*. New York: Rodale. A popular book with an eight-week course on mindfulness.

How Trauma and Burnout Overlap

Fried. The Burnout Podcast: A podcast from two burnout coaches, Cait Donovan and Sarah Vosen, who hone in on the many traumas that can lead to burnout and explore holistic approaches to address this.

Maté, G. with Maté, D. (2022). *The Myth of Normal*. Penguin Random House. A deep exploration into the way our society normalizes toxic stress and how this creates mental-health difficulties.

Everyday Burnout Conversations: A podcast by journalist and burnout coach Flic Taylor who interviews experts on their insight related to burnout, from growing up with alcohol-dependent parents to toxic work culture.

Thriving in a Team

Manual of Me: A website for reflective questions about your preferences and responses to stress, which you can share with colleagues or family members if you choose. See their website for more information: www.manualof.me.

Braune, G. (2022). *All That We Are: Uncovering the Hidden Truths About Our Behavior at Work*. Piaktus. A fascinating journey of case studies into various places of work by a psychotherapist. This gives you an idea of the invisible layers when there is tension at work and the psychology of interactions. This can help you get fresh perspective of any problems in your own place of work.

Specific to Health Professionals
You Are Not a Frog: A podcast by a physician, Dr. Rachel Morris, for burned-out health professionals. It features quick episodes with practical psychological tools in addition to longer interviews.
When Work Hurts: A podcast by a clinical psychologist, Dr. Paula Redmond, which discusses issues relating to burnout in healthcare.

Specific to Parents
Druckerman, P. (2013). *French Children Don't Throw Food*. Black Swan. An interesting book written by a mother and journalist who moves to Paris. It explores the way French people parent their children, highlighting the different boundaries and norms that might support them to feel less stressed.
Motherkind podcast with Zoe Blaskey: A relatable podcast hosted by a parenting coach that explores issues related to parenthood and well-being.
The Therapy Edit podcast: Hosted by psychotherapist Anna Mathur, it features a mixture of short solo episodes that give therapy tips, in addition to longer interviews, for overstretched parents.
Berry, B. (2020). *Motherwhelmed*. Revolution from home publishing. A book that deconstructs the invisible pressures in motherhood.

INDEX

Note: Page numbers with *asterisks* refer to diagrams.